Gerontological Nurse
Certification Review

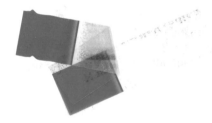

Meredith Wallace, PhD, APRN-BC, ANP, completed her BSN degree magna cum laude at Boston University. She earned an MSN in medical-surgical nursing with a specialty in geriatrics from Yale University and a PhD in nursing research and theory development from New York University. During her time at NYU she was awarded a predoctoral fellowship at the Hartford Institute for Geriatric Nursing. In this capacity she became the original author and editor of the series Try This: Best Practices in Geriatric Nursing. In 2001, she won the Springer Publishing Company Award for Applied Nursing Research. She was the managing editor of the *Journal of Applied Nursing Research* and is currently the research brief editor for the journal.

Wallace is the author of numerous journal articles and book chapters. She authored *Prostate Cancer: Nursing Assessment Management and Care* (2002), which won an *American Journal of Nursing* Book of the Year Award. Preceding this, she was the associate editor of the *Geriatric Nursing Research Digest* (2002), and she was the associate editor of the second edition of the *Encyclopedia of Nursing Research* (2006), both of which also won *American Journal of Nursing* Book of the Year Awards. She is a recipient of the Eastern Nursing Research Society/John A. Hartford Foundation junior investigator award. She is an adult nurse practitioner and currently maintains a practice in primary care with a focus on chronic illness in the elderly.

She is currently an associate professor at Yale School of Nursing, in New Haven, Connecticut. Her research interests focus on the psychosocial needs of men with prostate cancer, especially those undergoing active surveillance.

Sheila Grossman, PhD, APRN-BC, FNP, is a professor of nursing and specialty director of the family nurse practitioner track at Fairfield University School of Nursing. She graduated from the University of Connecticut with a BS degree in nursing, received her MS degree as a respiratory clinical nurse specialist from the University of Massachusetts Amherst, a postmasters degree as a family nurse practitioner from Fairfield University, and her PhD in professional higher educational administration from the University of Connecticut. She has multiple years as a clinician on a variety of medical, surgical, and critical care units and presently practices as a family nurse practitioner in primary care. She teaches pathophysiology and pharmacology, medical and surgical nursing, critical care nursing, and leadership and management to undergraduate students and advanced physiology and pathophysiology, leadership, and adult health to graduate students.

She is the coauthor of *The New Leadership Challenge: Creating a Preferred Future for Nursing,* which is in its third edition (2008) and has received an *American Journal of Nursing* Book of the Year Award for *Mentoring in Nursing: A Dynamic and Collaborative Process* (2007). She is the author of multiple chapters and journal articles on leadership, mentoring, gerontology, adult health, and other topics. Her research interests focus on symptom management in palliative care, leadership, and adult patient outcome studies.

Gerontological Nurse Certification Review

Meredith Wallace, PhD, APRN-BC, ANP
Sheila Grossman, PhD, APRN-BC, FNP

SPRINGER PUBLISHING COMPANY

New York

Springer Publishing Company, LLC
11 West 42nd Street
New York, NY 10036
www.springerpub.com

Acquisitions Editor: Allan Graubard

Production Editor: Julia Rosen

Cover design: Joanne E. Honigman

Composition: Apex CoVantage, LLC

11 12 13 14 15 / 10 9 8 7 6

Library of Congress Cataloging-in-Publication Data

Wallace, Meredith, PhD, RN.
   Gerontological nurse certification review / Meredith Wallace, Sheila Grossman.
      p. ; cm.
   Includes bibliographical references and index.
   ISBN 978-0-8261-0114-3 (alk. paper)
   1. Geriatric nursing—Examinations, questions, etc. I. Grossman, Sheila. II. Title.
   [DNLM: 1. Geriatric Nursing—Examination Questions. 2. Geriatric Assessment—Examination Questions. WY 18.2 W192g 2008]
   RC954.W254 2008
   618.97'02310076—dc22   2008009541

Printed in the United States of America by Bang Printing.

This book is dedicated to Mathy Mezey, PhD, RN, FAAN, professor of nursing education at New York University College of Nursing and director of The John A. Hartford Foundation Institute for Geriatric Nursing, for her lifelong love and passion for geriatric nursing excellence and her consistent recognition of certification as the benchmark for excellence in geriatric nursing care.

Contents

Foreword xiii

Preface xv

Chapter 1   Information for Taking the Certification Exam 1

Certification Exam Format 2

Detailed Test Content Outline 2

Total Number of Questions 3

Total Time 3

Obtaining the Application 3

Eligibility to Take the Exam 3

Scheduling the Test 3

What to Bring on the Day of the Exam 4

Time of Arrival 4

During the Exam 4

Receiving Test Results 4

Receiving Certificate and Pin 5

Hints for the Certification Exam 5

Chapter 2   Question Dissection and Analysis 7

Preparation Strategies 7

Review Content of Frequent Conditions
Experienced by Older Adults 9

Strategies for Analyzing the Questions 9

Clues to Memorizing Information 10

Two Different Ideas in One Question 10

Prioritizing 11

Conclusion 12

Chapter 3   The Aging Population 13

Demographics 13

Categories of Aging 14

Ageism and Myths Among Nurses and Other
Health Care Staff 14

Cultural Sensitivity 18

Theories of Nursing, Aging, Family, and Motivation 19

Nursing Theories 19

Aging Theories 21

Family Theory 22

Motivational Theory 23

Communication With Older Adults 23

Teaching-Learning Theories and Principles 26

Gerontological Nursing Today 27

Chapter 4 Assessment 29

History and Physical Exam Considerations 29

Health History 29

Physical Assessment 32

Normal Aging Changes 37

Cardiovascular System 37

Peripheral Vascular System 37

Respiratory System 38

Integumentary System 38

Gastrointestinal System 38

Urinary System 39

Sexual/Reproductive System 40

Sensory System 40

Neurological System 41

Chapter 5 Health Promotion 43

Levels of Prevention 43

Primary Prevention 43

Secondary Prevention (Screening) 44

Tertiary Prevention (Disease Management) 44

Barriers to Health Promotion Among Older Adults 44

Alcohol Use 44

Smoking 47

Nutrition and Hydration 47

Exercise 48

Sleep 48

Adult Immunization 51

Alternative and Complementary Health Care 55

Chapter 6   Environments of Care 59

Safety and Security Issues 59

    Falls 59

Use of Restraints 60

Hypo- and Hyperthermia...................................62

Relocation..62

Transportation..63

Territoriality and Personal Space 64

Community-Based Services and Resources..................65

Residential Facilities......................................66

    Skilled Nursing Facilities 66

    Assisted Living Facilities.............................67

    Continuing Care Retirement Communities..................67

Homeless Elders 68

Chapter 7   Spirituality and Death and Dying......................... 71

Principles of Effective End-of-Life Care 71

    Physical Dimension...................................72

    Psychological Dimension..............................72

    Social Dimension....................................75

    Spiritual Dimension..................................75

Advanced Directives 78

Hospice and Palliative Care 80

Grieving 81

Widowhood 82

Chapter 8   Acute and Chronic Physical Illnesses 83

Cardiac and Peripheral Vascular Problems 83

    Hypertension 83

    Congestive Heart Failure..............................84

    Angina and Myocardial Infarction 86

    Peripheral Vascular Disease...........................88

Respiratory Problems......................................89

    Pneumonia 89

    Influenza 90

Tuberculosis 91

Obstructive Airway Disease 92

Gastrointestinal Problems 92

Gastroesophageal Reflux Disease 92

Hematological Problems 93

Anemia 93

Genitourinary Problems 94

Urinary Tract Infections 94

Sexually Transmitted Diseases 94

Cancer 96

Prostate Cancer 97

Breast Cancer 98

Musculoskeletal Problems 98

Osteoarthritis and Degenerative Joint Disease 98

Osteoporosis 99

Metabolic and Endocrine Problems 100

Diabetes Mellitus 100

Immunologic Problems 101

*Human Immunodeficiency Virus/Acquired Immune
Deficiency Syndrome* 101

Neurological Problems 102

Parkinson's Disease 102

Cerebral Vascular Accident 104

Decubitus 105

Decubitus Ulcers 105

Sensory Problems 108

Common Eye Diseases 108

Common Ear Disease: Presbycusis 110

Chapter 9   Cognitive and Psychological Disorders 111

Introduction 111

Relationship of Depression and Suicidal Ideation 118

Dementia 119

Delirium 122

Chapter 10 Medication 125

Polypharmacy 125

Pharmacokinetics and Pharmacodynamics 126

Adverse Drug Reactions and Side Effects 128

Compliance Issues. 129

Chapter 11   Special Issues 131

Pain 131

Sexuality 133

Elder Neglect and Abuse 136

Chapter 12   Organizational and Health Policy Issues. 139

Advocacy for Older Adults 139

Health Care Delivery Systems 140

Reimbursement 140

Older Americans Act 141

Medicare and Medigap 141

Medicare Managed Care, Prospective Payment Systems,
and Other Medicare Systems 162

Medicaid 163

Long-Term Care Insurance 165

Veteran's Benefits 166

Chapter 13   Scope and Standards of Geriatric Nursing Practice. 169

Leadership and Management 169

Quality Improvement 171

Organizational Concepts. 172

Professional Development 172

Legal and Ethical Issues. 173

Regulatory Guidelines 173

Ethical Principles and Decision Making .173

Research 174

Evidence-Based Practice. 175

Posttest. 177

Index. 271

Foreword

For several decades, policy experts and healthcare professionals have made projections regarding the coming baby boomer bubble of an aging American population. The recent Institute of Medicine report, *Retooling for an Aging America: Building the Health Care Workforce,* details the dramatic changes in the size and composition of the aging American population and the challenges this will create for health professionals of all kinds. Those projections have come to fruition, creating an urgent need for health care professionals and nurses in particular to have a strong base of knowledge and skills in care of the older adult. Demographic realities will create a doubling of adults over the age of 65 in the very near term, adding to the rapidly increasing number of individuals in this country who are termed the oldest old. Amazingly, Hallmark Cards reports that annually it sells over 85,000 cards for centenarian birthdays.

The aging of America has created a dynamic and changing perspective on aging. Older adults are living longer while maintaining active and full employment, social, and community lives. However, this longevity is accompanied by a concurrent increase in chronic illnesses treated with sophisticated technological and pharmacological interventions. This enormously complex array of treatments creates the need for a health professional workforce that is prepared to meet the unique physiological and psychosocial needs of older adults. The unique skill sets that are required to provide safe, high quality and effective care to older adults are not intuitively acquired, but rather come only from a focused approach to developing new views and knowledge that will shape and define how care will be delivered to the older adult.

Unfortunately, despite the growth in the population of older adults, the nursing profession has not seen a concomitant increase in the proportion of the nursing workforce with a specialization in geriatrics. However, increasingly nurses and other professionals are seeking the specific skill sets necessary to deliver high quality care to older adults. Much of the enhanced focus on geriatrics comes as a result of the important and substantial support that has been made available to the nursing profession by the John A. Hartford Foundation. Through this support, an enhanced focus on both geriatric practice and research has blossomed in the profession and nursing professionals have increasingly sought the specific knowledge and skills necessary. As they seek this knowledge, they also seek the professional validation represented by certification by a national body as a specialized geriatric clinician. Certification is an external validation of competence to meet specific and important needs is the hallmark of excellence in nursing practice.

This new publication is an important addition to the resources available for nurses who seek certification as a geriatric clinician. This resource, designed for the generalist baccalaureate-educated nursing clinician who desires validation of expert knowledge and skills for care of the older adult, also recognizes the reality of practice. Generalist practice is almost uniformly geriatric practice. The preponderance of older adults in today's acute care facilities, long-term care settings, and communities should create an awareness among all nursing professionals that the knowledge and skills assessed through geriatric certification are a basic foundation for safe practice today.

In this book, the tools and clear presentation of information related to the actual testing process provide the learner with a framework for confidence as he or she prepares for the exam. More important, however, is the elaborate presentation of the certification content and the attention to the important physical and psychosocial elements of the human aging process.

The American Nurses Association Scope and Standards of Practice Statement expresses clearly the central role nurses play in protecting and assuring that safe and effective care is delivered. This statement notes: "Today as in the past, nursing remains pivotal in improving the health status of the public and ensuring safe, effective, quality care." This mandate for nursing to engage in safe, effective, high-quality care cannot be met for older adults absent a strong base of knowledge regarding the unique needs of this population. As nurses strive to engage in this level of practice, certification will validate our commitment to providing the best care possible. This book will enable nursing professionals to acquire certification as a geriatric specialist and provide them with the ability to achieve this important and professionally responsible goal.

Geraldine Bednash, PhD, RN, FAAN
Executive Director
American Association of Colleges of Nursing

Preface

The *Gerontological Nurse Certification Review* has been written as a reference and certification test review guide for registered nurses (RNs) preparing for gerontological certification. It is also a useful text for students who are studying gerontology, teachers preparing gerontology classes, and RNs working with older adults. The book presents information about preparing for the certification exam, a comprehensive compilation of content specific to gerontology, and a test bank of questions specifically developed for the RN preparing for certification in gerontology.

The book provides necessary step-by-step information for the candidate for certification to prepare and take the test in chapters 1 and 2. The remaining chapters 3 through 13 are organized according to the various topics of the blueprint of the Gerontological Nurse Certification Exam for baccalaureate and associate degree nurses. Chapter 3 focuses on topics specific to the aging population such as demographics, myths about aging, theories of aging and nursing, communication skills geared for the older adult, teaching-learning principles that work well with older adults, and the history of gerontological nursing. Chapter 4 describes the normal aging changes and questions referring to history and physical exam of older adults. Chapter 5 identifies the health promotion needs of elders such as nutrition, exercise, primary and secondary prevention strategies, and alternative and complementary health care practices used with older adults. Chapter 6 describes the environment, including safety and security, relocation, transportation, the importance of space, community-based resources, and residential facilities. Spirituality and dying are discussed in chapter 7 with regard to advanced directives, hospice and palliative care, and the grieving process. Chapter 8 describes the acute and chronic physical illnesses most frequently experienced by older adults. Chapter 9 discusses the cognitive and psychological disorders experienced by elders, including dementia, delirium, and depression. Common medications used by older adults along with discussions about polypharmacy, issues related to pharmacokinetics and pharmacodynamics, noncompliance, and adverse drug effects are covered in chapter 10. Special topics such as pain, sexuality, and elder neglect and abuse are discussed in chapter 11. Descriptions of health policy issues and organizations that advocate for older adults are covered in chapter 12. Finally, chapter 13 discusses the scope and standards of geriatric nursing practice relating to leadership and management, research, ethical and legal issues, and professional competency.

A posttest contains 514 test questions and correct answers covering all the various content areas. Readers can choose to take the comprehensive integrated test under simulated timed conditions or select parts of the test bank to take at different times scheduled for the convenience of the individual.

The importance of practicing psychomotor skills, communicating with others, and increasing experience with various competencies such as leading, delegating, organizing, and assessing is clear. Thus, practicing reading scenario questions and answering them is considered very important in achieving success with an exam. Research indicates that the more practice an individual has taking questions similar to the exam they are preparing for, the higher success rate they will achieve (Bonis, Taft, & Wendler, 2007; Griffiths, Papastrat, Czekanski, & Hagan, 2004). Moreover, with the increasing elderly population, exam success is essential to the availability of a nursing workforce educated in assessing and meeting the needs of older adults. The authors hope that all nurses who complete this preparation book will be able to gain valuable knowledge, validate their competency on the certification test, and improve their ability to deliver high quality care to older adults.

References

Bonis, S., Taft, L., & Wendler, M. (2007). Strategies to promote success of the NCLEX-RN. *Nursing Education Perspectives, 28*(2), 82–87.

Griffiths, M. J., Papastrat, K., Czekanski, K., & Hagan, K. (2004). The lived experience of NCLEX failure. *Journal of Nursing Education, 43*(7), 322–325.

Information for Taking the Certification Exam

The *Gerontological Nurse Certification Review* prepares registered nurses (RNs) to take the national Gerontological Nurse exam offered by the American Nurses Credentialing Center (ANCC). By obtaining gerontological certification, nurses gain power similar to board-certified physicians and advanced practice nurses. There is an incentive to become certified in one's area of expertise. Most institutions will apply certification toward promotion to the next staff level. Some institutions give a bonus or a differential pay raise for certification. If you are affiliated with a Magnet hospital that supports certification for professional development, you will be further recognized. Most importantly, certification is an excellent way to be recognized for expertise in a specialty area. It is highly likely your institution will reimburse you for the fee required to obtain certification status.

The purpose of this chapter is to explain:

- The ANCC testing format
- The application and scheduling of the test date for certification in gerontology
- General hints to improve your preparation for the exam

Certification Exam Format

The ANCC only offers a computer-based test in multiple-choice format with the option of choosing one of four possible answers. The test contains 150 questions and covers content knowledge and application of professional nursing regarding gerontology at an entry-level competency. The exam is developed from information from role delineation studies that measure the necessary knowledge and skills needed for competent practice in a specialty area such as gerontology (Stromberg et al., 2005). The purpose of the exam is to assess whether nurses are competent to assess the strengths of older adults in order to facilitate their highest quality of life and, when appropriate, a "good death." The ANCC updates the RN gerontology certification exam on a regular basis. A 75-question Practice Certification Examination and answers can be accessed at http://www.anfonline.org/ANF/geroexam.pdf. Completing the practice exam and reviewing your answers is strongly recommended.

Table 1.1 lists the 10 exam topic areas, the corresponding number of questions that are asked about each area, and the percentage of the test that correlates with each content.

Detailed Test Content Outline

This book is organized chapter by chapter according to the ANCC RN Gerontology Test Content Outline, which can be seen in detail at http://www.nursecredentialing.org/cert/TCOs/09Gero_TCO.html.

1.1 ANCC Domains of Practice

Topic area	Percentage of the exam	Number of questions
Aging as it relates to older adults	2%	3
Health issues	30%	45
Communication	8.67%	13
Nursing process	16%	24
Lifestyle, health changes, and vulnerability in older adults	16.67%	25
Education	3.33%	5
Health promotion and wellness	10%	15
Management/leadership	7.33%	11
Legal and ethical issues	4.67%	7
Research	1.33%	2

Note. Adapted from the ANCC Gerontology Certification Exam Content Outline, June 4, 2007. http://www.nursecredentialing.org/cert/TCOs/09Gero_TCO.html

Total Number of Questions

There are 175 questions on the test, but 25 of them are pilot questions and do not count toward one's score. There is no way to determine which of the 175 questions count for your test, so it is best to consider each question as carefully as you can. This is the standard approach for validating new questions and ensuring that they are reliable.

Total Time

The time allowed to take the test is 3.5 hours. If desired, test takers can take a 20-minute practice exam to become oriented to the computer system. This is highly recommended for all test takers. This tutorial can be reviewed by going to the ANCC Web site at http://www.anfonline.org/ANF/geroexam.pdf. Most people complete the exam in about 2.5 hours, but ANCC allows 3.5 hours to take the exam.

Obtaining the Application

Eligibility to Take the Exam

To take the certification exam, you must provide payment (see the ANCC Web site for details about the cost), a copy of your current unrestricted RN license, documentation that you have practiced full time as an RN the equivalent of 2 years, have a minimum of 2,000 hours of clinical practice in gerontology in the last 3 years, and the completed application. You must also provide documentation of 30 continuing education hours in the gerontology specialty that you have acquired in the last 3 years. In case you are ever audited, it is recommended that you maintain a file of your continuing education certificates. The application will request that you include a description of the continuing education course and how it is relevant to your geriatric practice if the title does not reflect gerontology clearly.

A *General Testing and Renewal Handbook* with testing information and an application can be accessed at http://www.nursecredentialing.org/cert/PDFs/examhandbook.pdf (American Nurses Credentialing Center, 2008). You can type directly onto the application and print it. The address to send the application is:

American Nurses Credentialing Center
PO Box 791333
Baltimore, MD 21279-1333

If you have any questions regarding the application, you can send an e-mail to certification@ana.org or call 1-800-284-2378 for further clarification of any information.

Scheduling the Test

The test is administered by Thomson Prometric Computer Testing Centers. To choose a location, first set up a date and time to take the computerized test on Prometric's Web site: http://securereg3.prometric.com. An authorization to test (ATT) will be mailed to you from the testing center. After you receive the ATT, call 1-800-350-7076 or visit http://www.2test.com and make an appointment during the 90-day eligibility time period stated on your ATT form.

Testing centers are located in every state and some sites in Canada, Puerto Rico, and Guam. You can schedule, reschedule, or cancel your appointment at the Prometric Web site, http://www.2test.com. Hours for testing are generally 8:00 A.M. to 5:00 P.M., and the testing center is open Monday through Friday. It is recommended that you schedule your test appointment as soon as you get your ATT in order to have the best opportunity of getting your desired day and time. If you decide to switch the date, time, or test site location, you need to follow the directions in the ANCC General Testing and Renewal Handbook located at http://www.nursecredentialing.org/cert/PDFs/ExamHandbook.pdf.

What to Bring on the Day of the Exam

You need to bring your ATT form and two forms of identification that match the name on your ATT. One form of ID must have your photo, and both forms must have your signature. One form must be your passport, a photo driver's license, or a photo government-issued ID card. You will not be admitted without the necessary forms of identification. You cannot take anything into the testing room. You will be provided with scratch paper and a pencil only. You will be given a locker to store your valuables, such as car keys and wallet.

Time of Arrival

Test takers *must* arrive 15 minutes earlier than the scheduled time. Failure to arrive early will cost you your appointment and require you to reapply.

During the Exam

There are no refreshment breaks. You can take a restroom break according to the instructions given at the testing center, but this time will be subtracted from your total time of 3.5 hours. You cannot ask any questions during the exam. When you complete the test, you cannot take the scratch paper from the testing room.

Receiving Test Results

All scores for the test are reported in the mail approximately 2 weeks after taking the test. The results will be in a standardized format with a pass or fail designation. Those who fail the exam will receive a diagnostic explanation for each of the content areas.

Receiving Certificate and Pin

Those who pass the exam receive a certificate, pin, and identification card that states ANCC certification. This certification is valid for 5 years. Information regarding recertification is available at http://www.nursecredentialing.org.

Hints for the Certification Exam

- There is no penalty for guessing, so it is recommended that test takers answer every question.
- The test covers general and frequently seen gerontological problems, not rare and exotic diseases.
- Be familiar with the common drugs used with older adults.
- Know the frequently occurring adverse drug events with older adults and be able to apply the Modified Beers Criteria.
- You should know the normal laboratory results for the diseases that older adults commonly experience.

References that are recommended by the ANCC regarding gerontology are available at http://www.nursecredentialing.org or by calling 1-800-284-2378.

References

American Nurses Credentialing Center. (2008a). *2008 General testing and renewal handbook.* Retrieved April 23, 2008, from http://www.nursecredentialing.org/cert/PDFs/examhand book.pdf

Stromberg, M., Niebur, B., Prevost, S., Fabrey, L., Muenzen, P., Spence, C., et al. (2005). Specialty certification, more than a title. *Nursing Management, 205*(5), 36–40.

2

Question Dissection and Analysis

Preparation Strategies

Preparing for a standardized exam usually causes some anxiety and fear. What is necessary to remember is that you are an experienced RN who has practiced full time as a registered nurse for the equivalent of 2 years or you have a minimum of 2,000 hours of clinical practice in gerontology in the last 3 years. Either way, you have some excellent expertise that you can draw on while preparing for this examination. You also have experience using the nursing process in many situations with older adults, so you already are experienced in

- Assessing
- Analyzing situations and prioritizing
- Planning
- Implementing the plan of care
- Evaluating patient outcomes

Everything that you do in your mind with the nursing process clinically in your practice you will be doing as you figure out and analyze the test questions.

A question may be designed to evaluate your assessment expertise or how you would prioritize and schedule care; a question may ask you to plan for a specific patient outcome given the data presented in the question, or you may be asked to choose the best way of caring for a condition. Some questions will depict a patient situation that needs evaluation. For all the questions, you will be critically thinking through the scenario using the nursing process. Your thought processes will mirror what you would have done in similar situations if you were at your work setting. Table 2.1 outlines the similar thought processes that occur when taking the exam and being in practice.

2.1 Performance in Clinical Practice Mirrors Thought Processes for Taking the Gerontological Nurse Certification Exam

Clinical practice	Analyzing test question
Assess the patient with a comprehensive review of symptoms during admission or episodically.	Take the data that are significant for patient assessment from the question stem and match them with the point of the question.
Analyze all of the data you collected in assessment and use it to plan the patient's care.	Take the significant clues from the question stem and prioritize all of the information so that you can make the most appropriate plan.
Plan the care necessary to meet the patient's needs. Remember to make priorities.	Review the stem of the question and choose the information that tells you the patient's diagnosis, current status, and whether there is a priority situation that needs immediate attention. Analyze this together and select from the possible answers the plan that best fits the patient's needs.
Implement the plan with a possible need for rescheduling some actions given the patient's needs.	Take the significant clues in the stem of the question that indicate what the patient needs now and in the future. Analyze all of the information and choose the sequence of actions that you would take if this was your patient in practice.
Evaluate the patient's outcomes with respect to the appropriate plan that was implemented.	Review the stem of the question and brainstorm about what you would be evaluating given the diagnosis and patient status. Choose the answer based on the standards of care and evidence-based practice you follow in clinical practice.

Review Content of Frequent Conditions Experienced by Older Adults

Some of the most significant content information necessary to competently care for older adults reflects assessing, analyzing, planning, implementing, and evaluating patient outcomes of conditions that older adults most frequently experience. These conditions are denoted as *red flag* problems. Red flag older adult problems are discussed in more detail in chapter 8, Acute and Chronic Physical Illnesses. You should review these areas carefully if you feel you do not have a competent level of knowledge regarding these conditions:

- Heart failure
- Hypertension
- Hypotension
- Coronary artery disease
- Myocardial infarction
- Peripheral vascular disease
- Pneumonia
- Emphysema
- Constipation
- Diarrhea
- Gastroesophageal reflux disease
- Peptic ulcer disease
- Diverticulosis
- Benign prostatic hypertrophy
- Incontinence
- Anemias
- Osteoporosis
- Osteoarthritis
- Hip fractures
- Diabetes mellitus
- Thyroid disease
- Dementia
- Confusion
- Depression and anxiety
- Cerebrovascular accident
- Parkinson's disease

Strategies for Analyzing the Questions

It is important to be familiar with the two parts of a question. The sentence or phrase that follows the question number is called the stem. The four possible answers are called distracters; only one of these is a correct answer. Many successful test takers cover the distracters with a piece of paper or their hand and read the stem of the question without looking at the distracters. After reading the stem, the test taker reflects on the question stem and thinks what comes to mind as the answer. Then the test taker reviews the distracters and chooses the one that is most similar to what had come to his or her mind after reviewing the stem. This process seems to be helpful to many successful test takers.

Additionally, test takers should realize that sometimes the correct answer to a question is not what they think is the most appropriate answer to a question. Test takers must assume that there is a "best" answer to each question, even though it may not be what they perceive to be the most appropriate answer. Timing oneself with practice questions is good preparation for a successful outcome on a standardized test such as this certification exam. The following section contains examples of challenging questions that may require some extra attention to correctly answer.

Clues to Memorizing Information

It is helpful when reviewing content before taking an exam to have certain methods of remembering information. For example, remembering the three Ps that indicate the three most common manifestations of diabetes mellitus—polydipsia = extreme thirst; polyuria = frequent urination; and polyphagia = extreme hunger—will assist in answering some questions. The following example illustrates the usefulness of the memorization technique of mnemonics.

EXAMPLE

A 77-year-old woman did not have an intact gag reflex in the neurological examination. The cranial nerve that is affected is

   a. V
   b. IX*
   c. XI
   d. X

Rationale for the correct answer—b: This is pure recall. It needs to be memorized by applying the information to a framework that you can remember. The gag reflex is absent in patients with damage to the glossopharyngeal nerve, which is the IX cranial nerve, because it is responsible for the afferent limb of the reflex. A mnemonic such as *On Old Olympus's Towering Top A Finn And German Viewed Some Hops* is helpful for memorizing the cranial nerves. Once you can remember the mnemonic to identify the 12 cranial nerves, then you can review the functions you have memorized for each cranial nerve.

Two Different Ideas in One Question

It is important to understand how some answer options contain two phrases or thoughts. These options really are sentences with two distinct points. Usually, the two phrases are connected by *and* or *but*. Both of these phrases must be true in order for this two-component answer option to be the correct one. One might be tempted to select a longer answer option, such as in the example on the next page with two true components. However, length does not mean that this answer is the best answer.

EXAMPLE

A 71-year-old woman has been taking steroids for asthma for 5 years. She presents with increased weight and puffy ankles, states that she feels hyperactive and "stressed," and complains that she has "increased hair in all of the wrong places." She is experiencing negative reactions to her treatment and is most likely developing

    a. Addison's disease
    b. Cushing's disease*
    c. Hyperaldosteronism
    d. Hypoaldosteronism

Rationale for the correct answer—b: Think of the difference between Addison's disease, which is a decrease in cortisol, aldosterone, and androgens, and Cushing's disease, which is an increase in cortisol, aldosterone, and androgens. One can easily remember that a person with Cushing's disease has the moon face, truncal obesity, and thin extremities. Given this information, one can analyze that if the patient has been taking steroids for asthma for 5 years, she would be puffy in her ankles and experience weight gain due to the excess aldosterone, have hirsutism, which means excessive hair in the "wrong places" due to increased androgens, and feel stressed and hyperactive due to the increased cortisol. So this woman has developed Cushing's disease.

Prioritizing

EXAMPLE

A 66-year-old woman shares with you that she is "eating like a cow" and "drinking everything in sight." She says this has been going on for a few months. When you ask whether she has also had urinary frequency, she responds that she has. As the nurse caring for her, you decide to call the attending physician to request

    a. Increased calories with the diet
    b. A nutritionist consultation
    c. A fasting blood sugar for the next morning*
    d. Stat blood work for a HgbA1C

Rationale for the correct answer—c: The three Ps are clearly spelled out by the patient and warn that she may be developing diabetes mellitus. The patient is not in danger of hypoglycemia or hyperglycemia given the symptoms she has reported; therefore, choosing answer c, a fasting blood sugar for the next morning, will be the most reliable answer and is your priority action. There is no sense changing diet or getting the nutritionist involved until it is known whether she has diabetes mellitus. HgbA1C is not a diagnostic measurement; it is a monitoring parameter, so there is no sense in using this presently.

Conclusion

Having reviewed these hints for analyzing questions and being aware of the most common comorbidities that older adults experience, it is recommended that readers review the content and answer the questions following each content area in the following chapters of this review book. Then it is a good idea to visit the ANCC Web site (http://www.nursecredentialing.org) and take the practice exams. Reviewing content that you have trouble with on the practice test will improve your ability to succeed on the gerontological nurse certification exam.

The Aging Population

Demographics

- Individuals aged 65 years can be expected to live an average of 18 more years than they did 100 years ago.
- The average life span or the average expected age of older adults is 83 years.
- Individuals aged 75 years can be expected to live an average of 11 more years, for a total of 86 years (http://www.health.gov/healthypeople).
- Older adults currently represent approximately 13% of the population. By the year 2030, they are expected to represent approximately 21% of the population.
- The increase in the number of older adults in the United States is known as the graying of America.
- The graying of America brings about multiple issues and concerns for society:
  - How a majority of older adults will be viewed as members of society
  - What resources will be available for older adults to live healthy and happy lives such as health care and housing

■ The average older adult has three chronic medical illnesses that have the potential to

■ Reduce quality of life
■ Increase health care costs

Categories of Aging

Dividing older adults into segments allows nurses to recognize the unique differences present in each stage of older adulthood and provide more effective care.

■ Adults aged 65 to 75 are the young-old.
■ Adults aged 75 to 85 are the old-old.
■ Those age 85 and older are the oldest old.
■ Those who are 100 years and older are centenarians.
■ With the life span continuing to increase, will we need more categories in the future?

People are living longer for a number of reasons.

■ Immunizations are available to prevent disease such as measles, mumps, rubella, chicken pox, and polio.
■ Annual influenza vaccination greatly decreases morbidity and mortality related to the flu and prevents complications of pneumonia.
■ Pneumonia vaccination is given to most older adults, especially high-risk patients—such as those with chronic obstructive pulmonary disease or splenectomies—and heart disease patients.
■ New diagnostic techniques assist in the early detection and treatment of disease.
■ Development of new medications to treat disease occurs daily.
■ Improved economic conditions and nutrition.
■ Stronger emphasis on health promotion has undoubtedly resulted in decreases in both illness and death among the population.

Ageism and Myths Among Nurses and Other Health Care Staff

Ageism is defined as a negative attitude or bias toward older adults, resulting in the belief that older people cannot or should not participate in societal activities or be given equal opportunities afforded to others. Ageism results in

■ Lack of medical care of older adults
■ Decreased access to services
■ The potential for altered dignity and respect
■ Abandoned hopes of contributing to society
■ Policies and care decisions that are inequitable for older adults

Older adults are combating ageism in a number of ways:

- Participating in large organizations that support older adults, such as AARP
- Demonstrating their continued and vast usefulness in society through volunteerism or grandparents' raising grandchildren who would normally rely on state aid for support

The foundation for ageism lies in the many myths of aging listed below:

Myth #1: Older adults are of little benefit to society.

- The rate of disability among older adults is steadily declining.
- Older adults are also mothers, fathers, grandmothers, grandfathers, aunts, uncles, brothers, sisters, friends, and professionals such as teachers, physicians, nurses, and clergy.
- Older adults are of great benefit to those with whom they maintain relationships and serve in these roles.
- Older adults are one of the nation's greatest and most underutilized resources in that they make up a large volunteer pool that saves states and governments funds in unpaid services.
- The number of older adults providing care to grandchildren continues to rise and supplies a significant amount of care that would normally fall on state government for support.

Myth #2: Older adults don't pull their weight in society.

- Older adults who receive Social Security and Medicare paid into the system from which they are now drawing.
- While many older adults retire, many others do not. In 2002, 13.2% of older Americans were working or were actively seeking work. A Gallup poll of 986 older adults reported that only 15% of older adults wished to retire, and the vast majority wanted to work as long as possible.
- Ageism in the workplace or sickness and disability may prevent older adults from working, although they may wish to.
- Older adults are also raising their grandchildren in record numbers because parents are
    - Ill (related to HIV and other chronic illnesses)
    - Abusive
    - Alcoholic or drug addicts
    - Incarcerated

Myth #3: Older adults are cranky and disagreeable.

- The continuity theory supports that individuals move through their later years attempting to keep things much the same and using similar personality and coping strategies to maintain stability throughout life. Thus, cranky old people were probably cranky young people, too.
- The average older adult has three chronic illnesses. Sickness—especially cognitive disorders—may alter an older adult's personality.

Myth #4: You can't teach old dogs new tricks.

- Older adults are never too old to improve their nutritional level, start exercising, get a better night's sleep, stop drinking and smoking, and improve their overall health and safety.
- Older adults are increasingly returning to school and increasing their level of education. Many colleges and universities allow older adults to attend classes for low or no charge. In fact, 17% of older adults have a bachelor's degree or more.
- Keeping intellectually active is regarded as a hallmark of successful aging.

Myth #5: Older adults are all senile.

- Memory losses are common in older adulthood, but are often falsely labeled as dementia.
- The development of dementia is not a normal change of aging, but a pathological disease process evolving from neurological, vascular, infectious, metabolic, or degenerative processes or through trauma.
- Dementia is a chronic loss of cognitive function that progresses over a long period of time.
- Alzheimer's disease is the most common cause of dementia among older adults, making up about half of all dementia diagnoses.
- There are approximately 4.5 million U.S. residents with Alzheimer's disease.

Myth #6: Depression is a normal response to the many losses older adults experience with aging.

- Recent research on depression indicates that there is more to the development of depression than the experience of loss.
- The nature versus nurture controversy has uncovered the role of neurotransmitters in the development of depression among older adults.
- Because of the many physiological changes in aging of older adults, this population is more susceptible to the effects of altered neurotransmission than any other age group.
- Depression rates are highest among older adults with coexisting medical conditions.

Myth #7: Older adults are no longer interested in sex.

- Because sexuality is mainly considered a young person's activity—often associated with reproduction—society doesn't usually associate older adults with sex.
- Recent surveys have shown that approximately 30% of older adults had participated in sexual activity over the past month.
- Nurses and other health care providers do not assess sexuality, and few intervene to promote the sexuality of the older population.
- Reasons for nurses' lack of attention to sexuality of older adults include lack of knowledge as well as general inexperience and discomfort.

Myth #8: Older adults smell.

- Although it is true that some older adults have bad personal hygiene, this is definitely not applicable to the majority of the population.
- The numbers of odor-producing sweat glands diminishes as people age, leading to less perspiration among older adults.
- Urinary and bowel incontinence—or the involuntary loss of urine and feces—occurs more commonly among older adults.
- Both urinary and bowel incontinence are pathological changes of aging that result in loss of bladder or sphincter control and are highly treatable.
- Increased attention to older adults' care will likely result in improved management of hygiene, incontinence, and associated disorders.

Myth #9: The secret to successful aging is to choose your parents wisely.

- This phrase from the popular work of Rowe and Kahn (1998) on successful aging leads society to believe that little can be done to slow the aging process, because it is all set out in a nonmodifiable genetic plan dictated by lineage.
- While genetics are responsible for some parts of the aging process, they become less and less important as older adults age.
- The role of environment and health behaviors significantly replaces the role of genetics in determining the onset of normal and pathological aging.
- Rowe and Kahn (1998) report that approximately one-third of physical aging and half of cognitive function is a result of genetic input from parental influences. That leaves two-thirds of physical aging and half of cognitive function to be influenced by environmental factors and health behaviors.
- Many older adults, especially centenarians (those who have reached the age of 100), report that the key to successful aging is to enjoy and get satisfaction from life.

Myth #10: Because older adults are closer to death, they are ready to die and don't require any special consideration at the end of life.

- This myth often leads health care professionals to offer less aggressive treatment for disease and to neglect essential components of end-of-life care for older adults.
- While death among older adults may occur after a long life, older adults are not necessarily ready for it.
- The end of life is a difficult time for many older adults, but it also presents the opportunity to complete important developmental tasks of aging.
- Nurses can play an important role in helping older adults to complete these developmental tasks that can make the difference between a good and a bad death.

Cultural Sensitivity

An unprecedented shift has taken place in the cultural backgrounds of the U.S. population, with the number of White older adults decreasing relative to increased numbers of Hispanic, African American, Asian, and other cultural groups.

- The United States currently functions under a health care system known popularly as the Western biomedical model.
- This model forms the basis of beliefs about health care in the United States.
- The model is based on scientific reductionism and is characterized by a mechanistic model of the human body, separation of mind and body, and disrespect of spirit or soul.
- Increased cultural diversity predicts a change in the manner in which traditional Western medicine is accepted in the United States and the need to understand other models of health and healing.
- Thus, new interest is being shown in the dominant healing practices of other cultures, including:
  - Herbal medicine
  - Acupuncture
  - Massage therapy
  - Biofeedback
  - Yoga
  - Tai chi
  - Stress reduction
- To fully understand how cultural shifts affect the way in which health care is accessed and accepted in society, it is first necessary to understand a few terms.
  - *Culture* refers to the way of life of a population or part of a population. Culture also reflects differences in groups according to geographic regions or other characteristics that comprise subgroups within a nation.
  - *Acculturation* is defined as the degree to which individuals have moved from their original system of cultural values and beliefs toward a new system.
  - *Ethnogerontology* is the study of the causes, processes, and consequences of race, national origin, culture, minority group status, and ethnic group status on individual and population aging in the three broad areas of biological, psychological, and social aging (Jackson, 1985).

Cultural competence is necessary for providing excellent nursing care for older adults of all cultural backgrounds. Purnell (2000) and Campinha-Bacote (2003) identify four stages of cultural competence.

- *Unconscious incompetence* is common to beginning nurses and is manifested by the assumption that everyone is the same.

- *Conscious incompetence* occurs as the nurse begins to understand the vast differences between patients from many cultural backgrounds but lacks the knowledge to provide competent care to culturally diverse patient populations.
- *Conscious competence* is the stage when knowledge regarding various cultures is actively obtained, but this knowledge is not easily integrated into practice, because the nurse is somewhat uncomfortable with culturally diverse interventions.
- *Unconscious competence* occurs when nurses naturally integrate knowledge and culturally appropriate interventions into practice (Campinha-Bacote, 2003).

The National Center for Cultural Competence was developed to increase the capacity of health care and mental health programs to design, implement, and evaluate culturally and linguistically competent services. The following steps are recommended:

- Examine personal beliefs and the impact of these beliefs on professional behavior.
- Acquire knowledge regarding commonly encountered population-specific health-related cultural values, beliefs, and behaviors. These practices are listed in Table 3.1.
- Aid in the development of culturally competent policies within the health care institution.
- Conduct competent cultural histories to determine the basis of the client's health care beliefs and practices.
  - Remember to ask about the patient's use of complementary and alternative therapy.

Theories of Nursing, Aging, Family, and Motivation

Nursing Theories

Nursing theory is comprised of a group of related concepts that guide practice. It is abstract (not measurable) and an essential component of professional knowledge base. Nursing theory contains four concepts:

- Person
- Environment
- Nursing
- Health

Nursing grand theories are abstract, connect and relate the four main concepts of nursing, are not generally measurable, and are not usually used to guide research. Examples of nursing grand theories are:

- Nightingale (1859)—enhancing the body's reparative processes by manipulation of noise, nutrition, hygiene, light, comfort, socialization, and hope.

3.1 Health Care Practices of Dominant Cultural Groups

Belief	Native Americans	African Americans	Asian Americans	Latin Americans
Origin of belief	Health beliefs and views of death predate modern U.S. history and vary by tribe.	African traditions are often integrated with American Indian, Christian, and other European traditions. Many African Americans grew up with little health care.	Classical Chinese medicine influenced traditions in Japan (Kampo), Korea (Hanbang), and Southeast Asia. In parts of Asia, Taoism and Buddhism have influenced the healing traditions.	Most Latino Americans practice the biomedical model, but among some elders, there may be reminiscences of other beliefs.
Focus of health	Strong emphasis on mind–body–spirit integration	Interaction of multiple causes of health as opposed to just physical causes	Characterized by a need for balance between yin and yang to preserve health. Interaction of basic elements of the environment (e.g., water, fire, earth, metal, and wood).	Religion is an important component of health.
View of illness	Sometimes seen as the result of an individual's offenses	Illness may be seen as the result of a physical cause—such as infection, weather, and other environmental factors—or from sin or great offense.	Illness is viewed as a threat to the soul.	Illness may be multi-dimensional in nature.
Components of care needed for healing	Use of herbs from native plants, spiritual healing, harmony with the environment. Ritual purification ceremony may be needed to improve health	Power of religion, Christian in some cases; and use of herbs, or "root working." The use of healers is rarely seen. Home remedies may be used. Experiences of segregation and memories of the Tuskegee Experiment may make older African Americans skeptical and distrustful of health care providers.	Herbs and diet may be used to unblock the free flow of qi (chi), or vital energy, through meridians in the body. Acupuncture, tai chi, moxibustion, and cupping are also used frequently. Illness is addressed not only through medicine, but also through social and psychological interventions.	An interaction of the biomedical model with complementary and alternative therapies provides the framework for health care.

Note. Gratefully adapted from the Collaborative on Ethnogeriatric Education. (2000). *Core Curriculum in Ethnogeriatrics.* Retrieved March 20, 2007, from http://www.stanford.edu/group/ethnoger/target.html

- Benner and Wrubel (1989) — caring as a means of coping with the stressors of illness; caring is central to the essence of nursing.
- Orem (1971) — caring and helping clients to attain total self-care.
- King (1971) — communication to help clients reestablish positive adaptation to the environment. Supports that the nursing process is defined as a dynamic interpersonal process between the nurse, client, and health systems.
- Watson (1979) — promoting health, restoring the client to health, and preventing illness.
- Roy and Andrews (1999) — identifying types of demands placed on the client, assessing adaptation to demands, and helping clients adapt. The adaptation model is based on physiological, psychological, and sociological adaptive roles.
- Neuman (1982) — assisting individuals, families, and groups in attaining and maintaining maximal level of total wellness by purposeful interventions. Stress reduction is the goal.
- Leininger (1991) — transcultural theory as a unifying domain for nursing knowledge and practice, providing care consistent with nursing's emerging science and knowledge with caring as a central focus.
- Henderson (1966) — focusing on the need to work independently with other health care workers assisting the client to gain independence as quickly as possible.
- Peplau (1952) — developing interaction between the nurse and client.
- Rogers (1970) — maintaining and promoting health, preventing illness, and caring for and rehabilitating ill and disabled clients through the humanistic science of nursing to help people develop into unitary human beings.
- Abdellah and colleagues (1960) — providing service to individuals, families, and society to be kind and caring but also intelligent, competent, and technically well prepared to provide this service; involves 21 nursing problems.

Aging Theories

Several categories of theories have been developed to describe why people age. Biological theories explain that the reason people age and die is because of changes in the human body (e.g., the Hayflick theory). Biological theories include

- DNA error
- Accumulation of free radicals
- Protein cross-linkage
- Wear and tear
- Cell division time-out
- Immunity
- Waste accumulation theory

Psychological theories support the idea that an older adult's life ends when he or she has reached all of his or her developmental milestones. Psychological theories of aging include those of

- Maslow—self-actualization
- Jung—self-realization
- Erickson—integrity versus despair

Moral/spiritual theories support the idea that once an older individual finds spiritual wholeness, this transcends the need to inhabit a body, and he or she dies. These theories include

- Tornstam's theory of gerotranscendence
- Kohlberg's theory of self-transcendence

Sociological theories explain that when an older adult's usefulness in roles and relationships ends, death occurs.

- *Disengagement theory* explains that as relationships change or end for older adults, through the process of retirement, disability, or death, a gradual withdrawing of the older adult is evidenced. Less engagement in relationships and social activities is seen, and while new relationships may be formed, these relationships are not as integral to life as previously necessary.
- *Activity theory* indicates that social activity is an essential component of successful aging. When social activity is halted because of death of loved ones, changes in relationship, or illness and disabilities that affect relationships, aging is accelerated and death becomes nearer.
- *Continuity theory* proposes that people age who most successfully carry forward the habits, preferences, lifestyles, and relationships from midlife into later life and predicts strategies people will use to progress into old age.

Family Theory

Family theory provides a framework for understanding human behavior and improving relationships in order to assist individuals, families, communities, and organizations work through major life issues. In older adulthood, major life transitions include

- Retirement
- Relocation
- Loss of spouse and other family members and friends
- Financial constraints

Effectively functioning families with good communication are critical to helping older adults make transitions smoothly and decreasing the risk of depression and other negative effects of stress. Poorly functioning family processes leave older adults at risk for ineffective coping. These families may benefit from family therapy as well as individual therapy.

- Key family theories include those of Freud and Bowen.

Motivational Theory

Motivational theory is generally associated with workplace employment and the desire to develop more effective employees.

- Herzberg's hygienic needs theory focuses on the need to avoid discomfort and achieve personal fulfillment through maintaining good relationships, work conditions, salary, status, security, and a satisfying personal life.
- McGregor's X-Y theory focuses on whether people are lazy or ambitious.
- Adams's equity theory focuses on patterns of fairness.
- McClelland's motivational theory centers on motivational power.

In relation to older adults, motivational theory can be more specifically applied to changes in behaviors needed to improve health, for example:

- Smoking cessation
- Alcohol withdrawal and abstention
- Nutritional changes
- Weight loss
- Exercise
- Sleep hygiene

Motivational theories support that it is critical to determine the motivational factor in order to change behavior. Thus, the determination of a critical end result and continuous feedback toward that result are important factors changing health behaviors among older adults. Researchers in motivational theory have identified the following potential motivators:

- Desire to avoid negative result of behavior
- Achievement of a goal
- Recognition of activity
- Health behavior itself
- Responsibility
- Advancement or progress
- Personal growth

Health promotion activities may be centered on these potential motivators to enhance compliance and success.

Communication With Older Adults

Communication with older adult clients is often complicated by many factors. Some factors that may result in a nursing diagnosis of impaired communication include

- Different languages
- Hard of hearing
- Dysphagia
- Dementia

In working with older adults, effective communication is essential and is the responsibility of the health care provider. Outcomes of successful communication include

- The client being able to communicate effectively with health care providers.
- The client utilizing alternative communication methods to convey his or her meaning.
- The client being able to correctly understand messages conveyed by health care providers.

Interventions to aid in effective communication include

- Assessing the client's receptive abilities—can the older adult understand what you are communicating?
- Assessing the client's expressive abilities—can the older adult communicate his or her needs and desires?
- Identifying the client's sensory impairments that affect his or her communication, such as

  - Hearing impairments
  - Aphasias
  - Visual impairments

- Facing the client directly and speaking slowly, clearly, and concisely
- Demonstrating the skill or activity that you would like to communicate to the older adult
- Using interpreter services as necessary
- Using paper, pencil, or computer communication when necessary
- Validating the client's understanding of messages by asking him or her to repeat what was said
- Being alert for nonverbal signs of behavior, especially in cognitively impaired older adults
- Providing older adult with yes/no choices
- Providing easy instructions in short, simple sentences
- Using physical cues and gesturing
- Limiting choices to reduce confusion

The Alzheimer's Association (2008) recommends a number of assessment questions and communication tips, which are displayed in Table 3.2. Assessment of specific receptive and expressive abilities is needed in order to understand the patient's communication difficulties and facilitate communication.

3.2 Tools to Assess Language Deficits and Facilitate Communication

Assess receptive abilities	How to facilitate communication
Can the patient understand a yes–no choice?	Ask simple, direct questions that require only a *yes* or *no* response.
Can the patient read simple instructions?	Provide instructions in a place that is easily visible to the patient.
Can the patient understand simple verbal instructions?	Use short, simple sentences. Use one-step instructions to enhance the individual's ability to process—for example, it's time to wash [smile; pause]; I will help you [pause and proceed]. Avoid slang, idioms, and nuances.
Can the patient understand instructions given with physical cues?	Use gestures. Model the desired behavior (e.g., eating). Be sensitive to the fact that, although the person may not understand words, he or she often can read your body language, sincerity, and mood.
Can the patient make a choice when presented with two objects or options?	Limit choices; too many options will cause confusion and frustration.

Assess expressive abilities	How to facilitate communication
Does the patient have difficulty finding the correct word?	If you are sure of the word the person is trying to say, repeat it. If you are not sure, then don't guess, because that will increase the person's confusion and frustration.
Does the patient have difficulty creating sentences or a logical flow of ideas?	Listen for meaningful words and ideas. Try to identify the key thoughts and ideas. Do not dismiss a person as "totally confused."
Does the patient curse, use offensive or aggressive language, or exhibit aggressive or combative behaviors?	Don't reprimand. Respond to the emotion, not the words. Validate feelings. Assess for unmet needs, including those related to misperceptions, hunger, thirst, toileting needs, pain, etc. (See Try This: Assessing Pain in Persons With Dementia.)
Does the patient avoid verbalization altogether or mutter meaninglessly in various tones?	Read nonverbal communication. Anticipate needs.

(continued)

3.2 Tools to Assess Language Deficits and Facilitate Communication (*continued*)

General Communication Tips

- If the patient's primary language is not English, determine whether he or she can communicate more effectively in another language; ask the family; and use an interpreter if necessary.
- Identify hearing and vision impairments; ask about prior use of assistive devices (hearing aids and glasses) and assure use of these devices in the hospital.
- Reduce environmental distractions that compete for attention when conversing with the patient.
- Approach the patient from the front, make eye contact, address the person by name, and speak in a calm voice.
- Talk first; pause; touch second, reducing the person's sense of threat.
- Avoid verbal testing or questioning beyond the person's capacity.
- Avoid using the in-room intercom, which may confuse and frighten the patient.
- Do not argue or insist that the patient accept your reality.
- Be aware of memory impairments in addition to communication difficulties. For example, if a patient's short-term memory is less than a few minutes, it is dangerous to leave the patient alone even if he or she seems to understand the direction, "wait here." Likewise, it is unwise to expect the patient to use a call light to get help. For patients with very impaired short-term memory, each encounter with a staff member may be perceived as the first encounter, even if the staff member just left the room and returned a few minutes later.

Note. From Alzheimer's Association. *Tips for Better Communication*. Retrieved March 24, 2008, from http://www.alz.org/living_with_alzheimers_communication.asp

Teaching-Learning Theories and Principles

Teaching refers to transference of knowledge, and learning results from an educational experience aimed at improving knowledge and skills or changing behaviors. Behaviorist theories focus on immediate and consistent positive feedback of good behaviors implemented as a result of the teaching-learning process. Negative behaviors associated with the process are ignored. Practicing the right behavior repeatedly is critical.

Cognitive teaching-learning theories focus on an active learning approach aimed at developing human insight. Goal setting and attainment are the underlying principles of this teaching-learning process.

Constructivist theories surround an engaging process that combines both behaviorist and cognitive strategies to promote effective teaching and learning. The foundation for learning is built on students' past experiences.

- Although many myths of aging lead health care providers to avoid teaching in this population, older adults are capable of gaining new knowledge and changing behaviors even at very advanced ages.

- Older adults have many heterogeneous educational experiences and learning styles that require individualization of teaching strategies.
- Identifying an older adult's learning style and individualizing one's teaching methods accordingly is important for successful teaching and learning to take place.
- Health literacy is defined as the degree to which an individual has the capacity to obtain, process, and understand basic health information and services necessary to make appropriate health care decisions.
- Low health literacy occurs frequently in older adults, who also tend to be those most in need of health services. Health literacy requires that older adults not only be able to read information, but understand what they are reading, hear instructions, calculate medications, and communicate questions.
- Low health literacy often impacts the ability of older adults to fully understand medication instructions and health interventions.
- Low health literacy disrupts a client's ability to effectively prepare for diagnostic tests, make follow-up appointments, and maintain health.
- Health literacy is a significant factor in noncompliance with health care treatments and medications.
- Clear communication has the capacity to assist those with low health literacy to maintain health.

Gerontological Nursing Today

With the increased population of older adults, there is a great need to increase the number of competent geriatric-educated nurses. Although nursing was the first profession to develop standards of gerontological care and provide a certification mechanism to ensure competence, gerontological nursing has been slow to gain recognition as a nursing specialty. While an increased number of nursing programs offer courses in geriatric nursing or integrate best geriatric nursing practices throughout programs, geriatric nursing is still not a popular specialty area among nursing students.

Some of the terms associated with nursing and the elderly are used interchangeably.

- Geriatric nursing refers to the nursing care of older people with health problems or those requiring tertiary care.
- Gerontological nursing includes health promotion, education, and disease prevention (primary and secondary care).
- Gerontic nursing, although not a commonly known term, encompasses both of these aspects of nursing care of older adults.

The American Nurses Association first recognized geriatric nursing as a specialty in 1966. Standards to guide the practice of gerontological nursing were first published by the American Nurses Association in 1976 and later revised in 1987 and 1995. Several organizations specialize in geriatric nursing.

- The National Gerontological Nursing Organization was developed in 1984 to support the growth of knowledge related to gerontological nursing science.
- The Gerontological Society of America, the American Society of Aging, and the American Geriatrics Society are multidisciplinary organizations that support aging knowledge and research.

References

Abdellah, F. G., Beland, I. L., Martin, A., & Matheney, R. V. (1960). *Patient-centered approaches to nursing.* New York: Macmillan.

Alzheimer's Association. (2008). *Tips for better communication.* Retrieved March 24, 2008, from http://www.alz.org/living_with_alzheimers_communication.asp

Benner, P., & Wrubel, J. (1989). *The primacy of caring: Stress and coping in health and illness.* Kent, OH: Addison-Wesley.

Campinha-Bacote, J. (2003). *The process of cultural competence in the delivery of healthcare services* (3rd ed.). Cincinnati, OH: Transcultural C.A.R.E. Associates Press.

Collaborative on Ethnogeriatric Education. (2000). *Core curriculum in ethnogeriatrics.* Retrieved March 20, 2007, from http://www.stanford.edu/group/ethnoger/target.html

Hartford Institute for Geriatric Nursing. (2000). *Try this: Best practices in nursing care to older adults.* New York: Author. Retrieved March 20, 2008, from http://www.hartfordign.org

Henderson, V. (1966). *The nature of nursing.* New York: Macmillan.

Jackson, J. J. (1985). Race, national origin, ethnicity, and aging. In R. Binstock & E. Shanas (Eds.), *Handbook of aging and social sciences* (pp. 264–268). New York: Van Nostrand Reinhold Company.

King, I. M. (1971). *Toward a theory for nursing: General concepts of human behavior.* New York: John Wiley & Sons.

Leininger, M. (1991). Transcultural nursing: The study and practice field. *Imprint, 38*(2), 55–66.

Neuman, B. (1982). The systems concept and nursing. In B. Neuman, *The Neuman systems model: Application to nursing education and practice* (pp. 3–7). Norwalk, CT: Appleton-Century-Crofts.

Nightingale, F. (1859). *Notes on nursing: What it is and what it is not* [With an introduction by Barbara Stevens Barnum and commentaries by contemporary nursing leaders. 1992, Commemorative edition]. Philadelphia: J.B. Lippincott Company.

Orem, D. E. (1971). *Nursing: Concepts of practice.* New York: McGraw-Hill.

Peplau, H. E. (1952). *Interpersonal relations in nursing.* New York: G.P. Putnam's Sons.

Purnell, L. (2000). A description of the Purnell model for cultural competence. *Journal of Transcultural Nursing, 11*(1), 40–46.

Rogers, M. E. (1970). *An introduction to the theoretical basis of nursing.* Philadelphia: FA Davis.

Rowe, J. W., & Kahn, R. L. (1998). Aging. *Aging, 10,* 142–144.

Roy, C., & Andrews, H. (1999). *The Roy adaptation model* (2nd ed.). Stamford, CT: Appleton & Lange.

Watson, J. (1979). *Nursing: The philosophy and science of caring.* Boston: Little, Brown and Company.

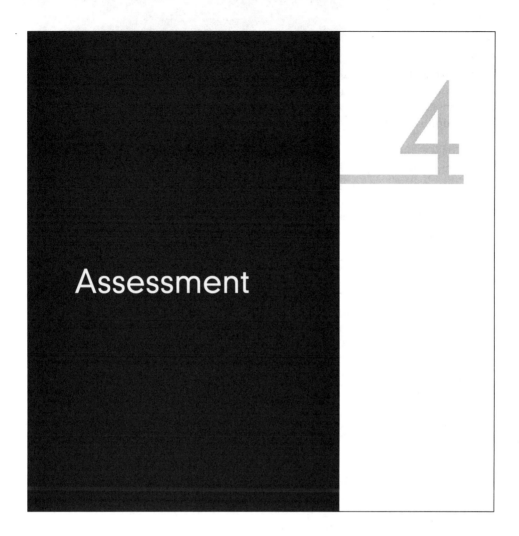

Assessment

History and Physical Exam Considerations

Health History

The health assessment always begins with a health history. This is usually the first meeting between the older adult and the nurse, and it marks the beginning of the therapeutic relationship. Nurses should focus on gaining the trust of older adult clients. A sufficient amount of time should be set aside for the health history so that the older adult does not feel rushed. Normal changes of aging result in an overall slowing down of response time. Older adults may have difficulty extracting dates and details from memory. There are many other challenges to getting a good healthy history from older adults, including:

- Age (older adults have a longer story to tell)
- Memory
- Tendency to underreport
- Communication difficulties

It is important to allow older adults time to think about their health history so as not to cause frustration about an inability to provide details surrounding former medical and surgical events. Older adults may withhold certain medical information from the interviewer because

- The information may be too distressing to discuss.
- The client may fear the consequences of their health problems. Memories of painful tests or the fear of a stressful diagnosis may cause the older adult to minimize symptoms.
- The client may fear being a burden on the health care system or on their children and thus hide or minimize symptoms of disease.

A health history includes

- Past medical history
- Past surgical history
- Cultural background
- Sources of social support
- Sources of financial support
- Occupation/retirement status
- Education
- Living arrangements
- Health promotion behaviors

  - Smoking
  - Alcohol use
  - Sleep patterns
  - Diet (use 24-hour recall)
  - Exercise
  - Use of herbal supplements

- Medications (including herbals and over-the-counter medications)
- Presence of common problems of aging

  - Dementia
  - Depression
  - Musculoskeletal disorders (osteoarthritis)
  - Sensory changes
  - Urinary function
  - Health literacy

Conduct a thorough review of systems.

- Cardiovascular system
- Respiratory system
- Peripheral vascular system
- Integumentary system
- Gastrointestinal system
- Genitourinary system
- Musculoskeletal system (ambulation)
- Neurological system (including senses)

Assess function and cognition as precipitating symptoms of illness in older adults.

■ A sudden decline in functional status or a change in ability to independently complete activities of daily living (bathing, dressing, toileting, eating, transferring, and ambulating) often signals the onset of physiological disease among older adults. The Katz Index (1970) is an excellent functional assessment tool that has been used widely in many health care settings to assess function among older adults.

■ Acute change in cognitive status known as delirium may be the first presenting sign of illness among older adults. This is true for both cognitively intact and cognitively impaired older adults. Because altered

4.1 The Mini-Cog and Mini-Cog scoring algorithm.

Administration

1. Instruct the patient to listen carefully and remember three unrelated words and then to repeat the words.
2. Instruct the patient to draw the face of a clock, either on a blank sheet of paper or on a sheet with the clock circle already drawn on the page. After the patient puts the numbers on the clock face, ask him or her to draw the hands of the clock to read a specific time.
3. As the patient to repeat the three previously stated words.

Scoring

Give 1 point for each recalled word after the clock drawing test (CDT) distractor.
Patients recalling none of the three words are classified as demented (score = 0).
Patients recalling all three words are classified as nondemented (score = 3).
Patients with intermediate word recall of one or two words are classified based on the CDT (abnormal = demented; normal = nondemented).
The CDT is considered normal if all numbers are present in the correct sequence and position, and the hands readably display the requested time.

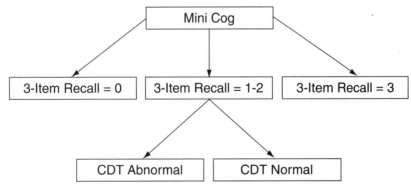

cognitive status is one of the more commonly occurring symptoms of disease among older adults, cognitive assessment using a valid and reliable instrument such as the Mini-Cog is appropriate (see Figure 4.1).

Physical Assessment

Following the health history and a complete review of systems, a head-to-toe physical examination should be conducted. This is how objective data are obtained in order to form diagnoses.

Evaluate the patient's vital signs.

- Temperature—response to infection among older adults varies greatly; some older adults respond to infections with elevated temperatures and others with aggressive infections showing no febrile response. Fever may be blunted among older adults because of

  - Diminished production and reduced response of pyrogens
  - Lower baseline temperature
  - Impaired immunity
  - Impaired ability to regulate heat and cold

- Pulse between 60 and 100 beats per minute—note irregular rhythms and follow up with electrocardiogram testing if necessary
- Respiration (12 to 18 breaths per minute)
- Measurements of height, weight, and body mass index (BMI) are essential to develop a baseline for further comparison of nutritional and hydration levels as well as bone loss. BMIs of less than 25 are considered ideal. BMI parameters are as follows:

  - Below 18.5 = underweight
  - Between 18.5 and 24.9 = normal
  - 25 to 29.9 = overweight
  - 30 and above = obese

- Blood pressure should be evaluated in the sitting, immediate standing, and 1-minute standing positions, especially if the older adult is taking antihypertensive medications. Decreases in blood pressure of more than 20 mmHg are indicative of orthostatic hypertension and require further evaluation. Blood pressure readings should follow the Seventh Report of the Joint National Committee on Prevention, Detection, Evaluation, and Treatment of High Blood Pressure (JNC-VII) blood pressure guidelines (see Table 4.1). It is helpful to keep in mind the following basic strategies for hypertension management.

  - Assess and manage blood pressure before it gets too high.
  - In people over age 50, systolic blood pressure is important and should be managed effectively.
  - Two or more antihypertensive medications are often necessary to maintain control.
  - Continued evaluation is often necessary, so maintenance of the therapeutic nurse-client relationship is essential.

4.1 JNC-VII Blood Pressure Guidelines

Blood pressure classification	Systolic blood pressure mmHG		Diastolic blood pressure mmHG
Normal	< 120	and	< 80
Prehypertensive	120–139	or	80–89
Stage I hypertension	140–159	or	90–99
Stage II hypertension	≥ 160	or	≥ 100

Note. From *The Seventh Report of the Joint National Committee on Prevention, Detection, Evaluation, and Treatment of High Blood Pressure*, by U.S. Department of Health and Human Services, National Institute of Health National Heart, Lung, and Blood Institute National High Blood Pressure Education Program, NIH Publication No. 04-5230, August 2004.

In addition to vital signs, the head-to-toe physical assessment includes evaluating the following:

- Skin

    - Hemangiomas
    - Liver spots
    - Harmless senile lentigines
    - Inflamed skin tags (skin projections)
    - Keratoses, precancerous, and cancerous lesions
    - Herpes zoster
    - Decubitus ulcers
    - Dryness

- Hair growth and nails

    - Uniformity
    - Diminished hair growth
    - Fungal infections of the nails

- Head and neck

    - Lesions or trauma.
    - Evaluation of the sclera for whiteness.
    - Notation of the arcus senilis (grayish arc surrounding the cornea and caused by lipid deposits on the cornea, not necessarily associated with high blood cholesterol).
    - Visual acuity.
    - Central vision (ability to see fine details, read, recognize faces).
    - Evaluate for cataracts and macular degeneration (the leading cause of vision loss among older adults) and refer to an ophthalmologist for follow-up of abnormal findings.
    - Identify the tympanic membrane and light reflex in the ear.

- Palpate nose for tenderness and signs and symptoms of infection.
- Evaluate mouth and teeth for deviations from normal and referrals made to a dentist for further management of mouth and tooth disorders.
- Palpate thyroid gland for enlargement and nodules.

- Heart and lungs

  - Evaluate the carotid arteries and jugular veins in the neck—they should be symmetrical, nonbounding, nondistended, and absent of bruits and adventitious sounds.
  - Inspect and auscultate the heart beginning at the apex. The first two heart sounds should be auscultated, and any adventitious sounds, murmurs, rhythms, and pulsations should be noted.
  - Murmurs (defective heart values) may be innocent (no associated signs/symptoms) or may be associated with

    - Shortness of breath
    - Enlarged neck veins
    - Dypsnea, perspiration on minimal exertion

  - Inspect lungs and palpate for tactile fremitus and equal expansion.
  - Percuss lung fields for areas of hyperresonance or dullness.
  - Assess peripheral pules, warmth and color in extremities.

- Musculoskeletal system

  - Assess ambulation.
  - Assess joint range of motion, tenderness, crepitus.
  - Begin at temporomandibular joint and proceed inferiorally to the ankles and feet.
  - Evaluate each joint, bone, and muscle group for abnormalities, tenderness, bilateral equalness, strength, and range of motion.

- Abdomen

  - Check for abnormal scars, pulsations, or distention.
  - Auscultate bowel sounds in all four quadrants.

- Genitourinary

  - Older women should continue to see a gynecologist for evaluation of breast and gynecological disorders common with aging.
  - Older men should undergo an annual examination for prostate enlargement or malignancies.

- Laboratory tests

  - Proper use of laboratory tests in evaluating older adults requires both knowledge of the normal ranges for age and the nurses' awareness of the client's health and medication history.
  - Laboratory tests commonly used in assessing older adults are provided in Exhibit 4.1.

4.1 Common Laboratory Tests Used To Assess Older Adults

Cholesterol: total cholesterol (TC), high-density lipoprotein (HDL), and low-density lipoprotein (LDL)

Normal Ranges

TC < 200 mg/dl
HDL > 50 mg/dl
LDL < 100 mg/dl

Tests the amount of circulating cholesterol levels. Good indicator for risk of cardiovascular disease, as well as to manage medications to prevent hyperlipidemia.

Complete blood count (CBC): hemoglobin (Hg), hematocrit (Hct), and white blood cells (WBC)

Normal Ranges

Men
Hg 13–18 g/dl
Hct 45–52%

Women
Hg 12–16 g/dl
Hct 37–48%
WBC 4,300–10,800 cells/mm^3

Tests for red blood cell (Hg, Hct, ESR) function and white blood cell function (leukocytes) to determine the ability of red blood cells to carry oxygen and white blood cell role in infection.

Drug assays (e.g., digoxin, dilantin, phenytoin, theophyllin, lithium)

See individual tests for reference ranges.
A collection of tests used to measure the level of certain medications in the body. Helpful in management of medication dosing.

Glucose and hemoglobin A1C (HgA1C)

Normal Ranges

Glucose (fasting) 70–105 mg/dl
HgA1C < 8%

Used to evaluate blood sugar levels and effectiveness of glucose management medications on glucose function among older adults.

Iron (Fe)

Normal Ranges

Serum iron 35–165 ug/L

Plays a role in hemoglobin and red blood cell function. Low iron is diagnostic for iron-deficiency anemia.

(continued)

4.1   Common Laboratory Tests Used To Assess Older Adults (*continued*)

International normalized ratio (INR)

Normal Range

INR 2–3

Tests body's clotting ability. Often used to evaluate response to warfarin therapy.

Kidney function tests (BUN) and creatinine

Normal Ranges

BUN 10–20 mg/dl

Men
Serum creatinine (CR) 0.6–1.2 mg/dl

Women
Serum CR 0.5–1.1 mg/dl
Commonly used to evaluate kidney function among older adults.

Liver function tests

See individual tests for reference ranges.
Used to evaluate normal and pathological liver functioning.

Prostate-specific antigen

Normal Range

PSA < 4 ug/L

Used to detect early signs of pathological prostate activity, such as benign prostatic hypertrophy or prostate cancer.

Thyroid function tests (T3, T4, TSH)

Normal Ranges

T3 75–220 ng/dl
T4 4.5–11.2 ug/dl
TSH 0.4–4.2 uU/ml

Because thyroid problems are prevalent among older adults, these tests are frequently used to determine thyroid function.

Vitamin assays

See individual tests for reference ranges.
Tests for function of vitamins in the body, such as vitamin X. Vitamins play an essential role in all bodily system functions.

Normal Aging Changes

Normal changes of aging are sometimes considered to be inevitable and irreversible. However, there is a great deal of variability in the age-related changes that occur among older adults. Individual aging is influenced by many factors that are both preventable and reversible. It is of critical importance for nurses to understand the normal physiological changes associated with aging. In so doing, nurses will be capable of differentiating these changes from abnormal or pathological organ system changes. These changes are discussed below, along with necessary nursing interventions.

Cardiovascular System

- The heart becomes larger and occupies more space in the chest.
- There is a reduction in the amount of functional muscle mass of the heart.
- There is a decreased amount of blood that is pumped throughout the circulatory system.
- More adventitious S4 heart sounds are evident.
- Premature contractions and arrhythmias may occur.
- Blood flow is slower.
- Wounds heal slower, impacts medication, metabolism, and distribution.
- Older adults often experience a low diastolic blood pressure.
- Older adults often experience an increased pulse pressure.
- While changes may be normal, they may also be indicative of cardiomyopathy, which warrants further cardiovascular assessment.
- Provide patient teaching regarding the role of exercise to ultimately reduce strain on the heart and blood pressure.
- Heart murmurs (S4) may require further tests to determine their effect.
- Fatigue, shortness of breath (SOB) and dyspnea on exertion (DOE), dizziness, chest pain, headache, sudden weight gain, and changes in cognitive function or cognition require full assessment.
- The time of effectiveness may take longer when giving meds.
- Low diastolic pressure is a risk for cerebrovascular accidents or strokes.

Peripheral Vascular System

- Increase in the peripheral vascular resistance (blood has a hard time returning to the heart and lungs).
- Valves in the veins don't function efficiently and form (nonpathological) edema.
- Inform patient that age, diet, genetics, and lack of exercise can transform nonpathological to pathological (atherosclerosis and arteriosclerosis), which can result in cardiovascular disease (CVD).
- Monitor older adults' cholesterol levels with lowering agents to prevent atherosclerosis and arteriosclerosis.
- Inform patients that exercise can lower cholesterol levels.
- Discuss the right medication, exercise program, and diet for the patient as a means to slow the progression of cardiac changes.

Respiratory System

- Vital respiratory capacity decreases.
- Lungs lose elasticity.
- Loss of water and calcium in bones causes the thoracic cage to stiffen.
- Amount of cilia lining system decreases.
- Cough reflex decreases.
- Auscultating sounds is difficult, so it must be done on all lung fields in a quiet environment.
- Inform patient that pollution and smoking worsen the cilia, so smoking cessation interventions might be necessary in the form of

  - Behavioral management classes
  - Support groups
  - Nicotine replacement therapies
  - Antidepression medications (Wellbutrin™)

- Implement interventions for older adults at risk for choking.
- Frequently assess respiratory function.
- Encourage regular exercise.

Integumentary System

- Skin becomes thinner and more fragile.
- Skin is dry and loses elasticity (wrinkles).
- Sweat glands lessen, which leads to less perspiration.
- Subcutaneous fat and muscular layers begin to diminish, which results in less padding and bruising more easily.
- Dryness is common.
- Skin tears are common.
- Fingernails and toenails become thick and brittle.
- Hair becomes gray, fine, and thin.
- Facial hair may develop on women.
- Body hair decreases on men and women.
- Promote the use of sun block, and tell patients to avoid overexposure to sun.
- Avoid the use of soaps that dry the skin and use lotion after bathing.
- Protect high-risk areas such as elbows and heels with padding.
- Refer patient to a podiatrist for effective foot care.
- Help older adults maintain their personal appearance.

Gastrointestinal System

- Inflamed gums, periodontal disease, sensitive teeth, and tooth loss are common due to lack of adequate fluoride and mouth care in younger years.
- Decreased peristalsis of esophagus, making food more difficult to swallow.

- Decreased gut motility, gastric acid production, and absorption of nutrients.
- Difficulty evacuating wastes (constipation).

  - Assess older adult's ability to chew.
  - Refer older adult for further oral evaluation if necessary.
  - Assist older adults in making changes in their eating habits.
  - Assess nutritional health frequently.
  - Encourage older adults to drink fluids.
  - Add bulk and fiber to diet.
  - Promote exercise.
  - Enemas and laxative medications may be given in severe situations.
  - Implement bowel habit training programs when necessary.
  - In severe cases, surgery may be appropriate to enhance ingestion and digestion of nutrients.

- Fecal impaction (primary cause of fecal incontinence) caused by

  - Polypharmacy (calcium channel blockers, iron)
  - Narcotic use
  - Immobility
  - Reduced fluid intake
  - Three Ds (delirium, depression, and dementia)

- Involuntary leakage of liquid stool (fecal incontinence) caused by

  - Loss of sphincter control
  - Decreased mobility
  - Decreased sensation in anal column

- Complications of fecal incontinence

  - Stigmatization
  - Social isolation
  - Depression
  - Fall risks
  - Skin breakdown

Urinary System

- Kidneys experience a loss of nephrons and glomeruli.
- Bladder tone and volume capacity decrease.
- Incontinence is not a normal aging change but often occurs in response to normal changes. Types of urinary incontinence include

  - Stress
  - Urge
  - Overflow
  - Transient

- Risk factors for incontinence include

  - Immobility
  - Impaired cognition

- Medication
- Constipation
- Diabetes
- Stroke

- Assess for urinary incontinence complications such as

  - Falls
  - Skin irritation
  - Social isolation
  - Depression

- Teach Kegel exercises when appropriate.
- Implement voiding schedules when necessary.

Sexual/Reproductive System

- There is an overall decrease in testosterone in men, and estrogen, progesterone, and androgen in women.
- Conduct sexual assessments.
- Help older adults feel comfortable when discussing sexuality.
- Women

  - Follicular depletion occurs in the ovaries.
  - Natural breast tissue is replaced by fatty tissue.
  - Labia shrink.
  - Vaginal lubrications decrease.
  - Shortening and narrowing of the vagina occur.
  - Strength of orgasmic contraction diminishes.
  - Orgasmic phase is decreased.
  - Artificial vaginal lubricants may help to compensate for normal aging changes.

- Men

  - Increased length of time may be needed for erections and ejaculation.
  - Inform men to increase the time between erections.
  - Discuss availability of oral erectile agents.

Sensory System

- Vision

  - Visual acuity declines.
  - Ability of pupil to constrict in response to stimuli decreases.
  - Peripheral vision declines.
  - Presbyopia is common, resulting from a loss of elasticity in the lens of the eye and leading to a decrease in the ability of the lens to refocus on near objects and light.
  - Lens of the eye often becomes yellow.

- Arcus senilus (ring around the cornea) may appear.
- Make sure older adults have a baseline eye assessment early in older adulthood and follow-up eye exams yearly.

- Hearing

  - Amount of hard cerumen increases.
  - Altered hearing is common.
  - Wax removal may be necessary.
  - Presbycusis is common, resulting from a gradual loss of high-frequency sensory neurons that conduct hearing.

- Taste and smell

  - 30% of taste buds diminish.
  - Obtain a thorough history of taste and smell sensations.
  - Conduct physical examination of the nose and mouth.
  - Obtain a thorough diet history.
  - Implement diet interventions to avoid overcompensation with sweet and salty foods.

Neurological System

- Total brain weight decreases.
- There is a shift in the proportion of gray matter to white matter.
- There is a loss of neurons.
- There is an increase in the number of senile plaques.
- Blood flow to the cerebrum decreases.
- Mild memory loss is common, but cognitive impairment is not a normal change of aging.
- Help older adults maintain an active body and mind.
- Encourage older adults to participate in cognitive activities.

References

Borson, S., Scanlan, J., Brush, M., Vitallano, P., & Dokmak, A. (2000). The Mini-Cog: A cognitive "vital signs" measure for dementia screening in multi-lingual elderly. *International Journal of Geriatric Psychiatry, 15*(11), 1021–1027.

Katz, S., Dow, T. D., Cash, H. R., & Grotz, R. C. (1970). Progress in the development of the index of ADL. *The Gerontologist, 10*(1), 20–30.

U.S. Department of Health and Human Services, National Institute of Health National Heart, Lung, and Blood Institute National High Blood Pressure Education Program. (2004, August). *The seventh report of the Joint National Committee on Prevention, Detection, Evaluation, and Treatment of High Blood Pressure.* NIH Publication No. 04-5230.

Health Promotion

Pathological changes of aging may result from poor health practices acquired early in life that continue into older adulthood. The Centers for Disease Control (2004) report that, in 2000, the most common causes of death in the United States were tobacco use, poor diet, lack of physical activity, alcohol consumption, and microbial agents. Despite their advanced age, older adults may still benefit from health promotion activities, even in their later years. In fact, health promotion is as important in older adulthood as it is in childhood. Older adults are never too old to improve their nutritional level, start exercising, get a better night's sleep, and improve their overall health and safety.

Levels of Prevention

Primary Prevention

Primary prevention involves measures to prevent an illness or disease from occurring and includes

- Smoking cessation
- Limited alcohol consumption
- Good nutrition
- Exercise
- Adequate sleep
- Safe lifestyles
- Updated immunizations

Secondary Prevention (Screening)

Secondary prevention refers to methods and procedures to detect the presence of disease in the early stages so that effective treatment and cure are more likely. Routine mammograms, hypertension screening, and prostate specific antigen blood tests are a few examples of this type of screening.

Strategies for detecting disease at an early stage involve annual physical examinations; laboratory blood tests for tumor markers, cholesterol, and other highly treatable illnesses; and diagnostic imaging for the presence of internal disease. Secondary disease-specific early detection guidelines are listed in Table 5.1.

Tertiary Prevention (Disease Management)

Tertiary prevention is needed after the disease or condition has been diagnosed and treated in an attempt to return the client to an optimum level of health and wellness despite the disease or condition. Physical, occupational, and speech pathology services following a cerebrovascular accident are typical examples of tertiary prevention strategies.

Barriers to Health Promotion Among Older Adults

- Misconceptions about the benefits of health promotion for older adults
- Separating the normal changes of aging from pathological illness
- Motivation to change (see motivational theories in chapter 3)
- Lack of reimbursement for health promotion behavior

Alcohol Use

Alcohol dependence and alcoholism has the potential for great consequences among older adults, including negative effects on

- Function
- Cognition
- Health
- Quality of life

5.1 Secondary Prevention Strategies for Older Adults

Intervention Considered and
Recommended for the Periodic
Health Examination

Leading Cause of Death
  Heart diseases
  Malignant neoplasm (lung, colorectal, breast)
  Cerebrovascular diseases
  Chronic obstructive pulmonary diseases
  Pneumonia and influenza

Interventions for the general population

Screening
Blood pressure
Height and weight
Fecal occult blood test[a] and/or
  sigmoidoscopy
Mammogram and clinical breast exam[b]
  (women ≤ 69 years)
Pap test (women)[c]
Vision screening
Assess for hearing impairment
Assess for problem drinking

Counseling
Substance Use
Tobacco cessation
Avoid alcohol/drug use while driving,
  swimming, boating, etc.[d]

Diet and Exercise
Limit fat and cholesterol; maintain caloric
  balance; emphasize grains, fruits, veg-
  etables
Adequate calcium intake (women)
Regular physical activity[d]

Injury prevention
Lap and shoulder belts
Motorcycle and bicycle helmets[d]
Fall prevention[d]
Safe storage or removal of firearms[d]
Smoke detectors[d]
Set hot water heater to 130°F or below[d]
CPR training for household members

Dental health
Regular visits to dental care provider[d]
Floss, brush with fluoride toothpaste daily[d]

Sexual behavior
STD prevention: avoid high-risk sexual
  behavior;[d] use condoms

Immunizations
Pneumococcal vaccine
Influenza
Tetanus-diphtheria (Td) boosters

Chemoprophylaxis
Discuss hormone prophylaxis, for
  menopausal women

Interventions for high-risk populations

Institutionalized persons

Chronic medical conditions: TB contacts;
  low income; immigrants; alcoholics
Persons 75 years or older or persons 70
  years and older with risk factors for falls
Cardiovascular disease risk factors
Family history of skin cancer; nevi; fair
  skin, eyes, or hair

Potential interventions (See detailed high-
  risk [HR] definitions)
PPD (HR1); hepatitis A vaccine (HR2);
  amantadine/rimantadine (HR4)
PPD (HR1)
Fall prevention intervention (HR5)
Consider cholesterol screening (HR8)
Avoid excess and midday sun, use protective
  clothing[d] (HR7)

(continued)

5.1 Secondary Prevention Strategies for Older Adults (*continued*)

Native Americans/Alaska Natives	PPD (HR1); hepatitis A vaccine (HR2)
Travelers to developing countries	Hepatitis A vaccine (HR2); hepatitis B vaccine (HR8)
Blood product recipients	HIV screen (HR3); hepatitis B vaccine (HR8)
High-risk sexual behavior	Hepatitis A vaccine (HR2); HIV screen (HR3); hepatatis B vaccine (HR8); RPR/VDRL HR9)
Injection or street drug use	PPD (HR1); hepatitis A vaccine (HR2); HIV screen (HR3); hepatitis B vaccine (HR8); RPR/VDRL (HR9); advice to reduce infection risk (HR10)
Health care/lab workers	PPD (HR1); hepatitis A vaccine (HR2) amantadine/rimantadine (HR4); hepatitis B vaccine (HR8)
Persons susceptible to varicella	Varicella vaccine (HR11)

ᵃ Annually.
ᵇ Mammogram every 1 to 2 years, mammogram every 1 to 2 years with annual clinical breast exams.
ᶜ All women who have been sexually active and who have a cervix: at least every three years. Consider discontinuation of testing after age 65 if previous regular screening yielded consistently normal results.
ᵈ The ability of clinician counseling to influence this behavior is unproven.
Note. Adapted from *Guide to Clinical Preventive Services*, by U.S. Department of Health and Human Services Centers for Medicare & Medicaid Services, 2007. Retrieved March 23, 2008, from http://odphp. osophs.dhhs.gov/pubs/guidecps/PDF/Frontmtr.pdf

Alcohol use is difficult to assess among older adults.

- Symptoms of alcohol use among older adults include alteration in mental status and function, which may mimic the symptoms of delirium, dementia, or depression.
- Older adults are usually no longer in the workforce, where the daily performance failures that are common with alcohol usage are often detected.

Alcoholism is a greater problem for older adults because older adults are not able to physiologically detoxify and excrete alcohol as effectively as younger people. Assessment of alcohol use may be most effectively accomplished using an instrument such as the CAGE questionnaire.

- Have you ever tried to **C**ut down on your drinking?
- Do you become **A**nnoyed when others ask you about drinking?
- Do you ever feel **G**uilty about your drinking?
- Do you ever use alcohol in the morning, as an **E**ye-opener?

Older adults with alcohol problems who receive treatment are capable of achieving positive health outcomes. In fact, when older adults receive effective treatment for their alcoholism, their prognosis is much better than it is for their younger counterparts. When alcohol abuse is suspected among older adults, it is necessary to refer them immediately to an appropriate program for effective treatment—such as Alcoholics Anonymous or an in- or outpatient detoxification and treatment program. Special treatment considerations should be applied to older adults during acute alcohol withdrawal related to normal and pathological aging changes.

Smoking

Cigarette smoking has multiple harmful effects on older adults, including, but not limited to, cardiovascular and respiratory disease and cancer. The current cohorts of older adults are among the first people who have potentially smoked throughout their entire adult lives. It is possible for older adults to experience the benefits of smoking cessation even in old age. It is important to note that older adults may be more motivated to quit smoking than their younger counterparts because they are likely to experience some of the damage that smoking has caused. Smoking cessation interventions include

- Behavioral management classes
- Support groups
- Nicotine replacement therapies
- Antidepression medications (Wellbutrin™)

Nutrition and Hydration

It is estimated that approximately 20% of older adult diets are inadequate. The many risk factors for nutrition among older adults include the following:

- Normal changes of aging place older adults at a higher risk for nutritional deficiencies
- Pathological diseases
- Decreases in smell, vision, and taste and the high frequency of dental problems
- Lifelong eating habits, such as a diet high in fat and cholesterol
- Diminishing senses of taste and smell result in less desire to eat and may lead to malnutrition
- Limited income
- Lack of transportation to purchase food
- Social isolation

Failure to thrive (FTT) is a syndrome used to describe clients who experience malnutrition in the absence of an explanatory medical diagnosis. FTT is often found with

- Dehydration
- Impaired cognition

- Dementia
- Impaired ambulation
- Difficulty with at least two activities of daily living
- Neglect

Nutritional assessment might use

- 24-hour recall
- Nutritional assessment forms (see Figure 5.1)

Interventions to promote nutrition include

- Patient teaching and reinforcements regarding good nutrition (see chapter 3 for a discussion of the theories and principles of teaching and learning)

  - A suggested resource is the MyPyramid food guide (see Figure 5.2)

Exercise

The role of regular exercise in promoting health and preventing disease cannot be sufficiently emphasized. Regular exercise results in

- Reduced constipation
- Improved sleep
- Lower blood pressure
- Lower cholesterol levels
- Improved digestion
- Weight loss
- Enhanced opportunities for socialization
- Improved pain control
- Increased temperature control in response to environmental changes
- Reduced risk of hypothermia

Despite the many benefits of exercise among older adults, the amount of exercise generally decreases as one ages.

Interventions to promote exercise include helping older adults to choose an exercise program that they enjoy and in which they are motivated to participate. Sample exercise programs include

- Walking
- Aquacise
- Strength training
- Yoga

Sleep

The inability to fall asleep and to sleep through the night are among the most frequent complaints of older adults. Many older adults report difficulty falling

5.1 Mini Nutritional Assessment.

Mini Nutritional Assessment
MNA®

Last name:		First name:		Sex:		Date:
Age:	Weight, kg:		Height, cm:		I.D. Number:	

Complete the screen by filling in the boxes with the appropriate numbers.
Add the numbers for the screen. If score is 11 or less, continue with the assessment to gain a Malnutrition Indicator Score.

Screening

A Has food intake declined over the past 3 months due to loss of appetite, digestive problems, chewing or swallowing difficulties?
0 = severe loss of appetite
1 = moderate loss of appetite
2 = no loss of appetite ☐

B Weight loss during the last 3 months
0 = weight loss greater than 3 kg (6.6 lbs)
1 = does not know
2 = weight loss between 1 and 3 kg (2.2 and 6.6 lbs)
3 = no weight loss ☐

C Mobility
0 = bed or chair bound
1 = able to get out of bed/chair but does not go out
2 = goes out ☐

D Has suffered psychological stress or acute disease in the past 3 months
0 = yes   2 = no ☐

E Neuropsychological problems
0 = severe dementia or depression
1 = mild dementia
2 = no psychological problems ☐

F Body mass index (BMI) (weight in kg) / (height in m)^2
0 = BMI less than 19
1 = BMI 19 to less than 21
2 = BMI 21 to less than 23
3 = BMI 23 or greater ☐

Screening score (subtotal max. 14 points) ☐ ☐
12 points or greater   Normal – not at risk – no need to complete assessment
11 points or below   Possible malnutrition – continue assessment

Assessment

G Lives independently (not in a nursing home or hospital)
0 = no   1 = yes ☐

H Takes more than 3 prescription drugs per day
0 = yes   1 = no ☐

I Pressure sores or skin ulcers
0 = yes   1 = no ☐

J How many full meals does the patient eat daily?
0 = 1 meal
1 = 2 meals
2 = 3 meals ☐

K Selected consumption markers for protein intake
• At least one serving of dairy products
(milk, cheese, yogurt) per day   yes ☐   no ☐
• Two or more servings of legumes
or eggs per week   yes ☐   no ☐
• Meat, fish or poultry every day   yes ☐   no ☐
0.0 = if 0 or 1 yes
0.5 = if 2 yes
1.0 = if 3 yes ☐ . ☐

L Consumes two or more servings of fruits or vegetables per day?
0 = no   1 = yes ☐

M How much fluid (water, juice, coffee, tea, milk) is consumed per day?
0.0 = less than 3 cups
0.5 = 3 to 5 cups
1.0 = more than 5 cups ☐ ☐

N Mode of feeding
0 = unable to eat without assistance
1 = self-fed with some difficulty
2 = self-fed without any problem ☐

O Self view of nutritional status
0 = views self as being malnourished
1 = is uncertain of nutritional state
2 = views self as having no nutritional problem ☐

P In comparison with other people of the same age, how does the patient consider his/her health status?
0.0 = not as good
0.5 = does not know
1.0 = as good
2.0 = better ☐ ☐

Q Mid-arm circumference (MAC) in cm
0.0 = MAC less than 21
0.5 = MAC 21 to 22
1.0 = MAC 22 or greater ☐ ☐

R Calf circumference (CC) in cm
0 = CC less than 31   1 = CC 31 or greater ☐

Assessment (max. 16 points) ☐ ☐ ☐

Screening score ☐ ☐

Total Assessment (max. 30 points) ☐ ☐ ☐

Malnutrition Indicator Score
17 to 23.5 points   at risk of malnutrition ☐
Less than 17 points   malnourished ☐

Note. The Mini Nutritional Assessment and MNA have been developed by and are trademarks owned by Société de Produtis Nestlé. © Nestlé, 1994, Revision 2006. N67200 12/99 10M
Sources: Overview of the MNA®: Its History and Challenges, by B. Vellas, H. Villars, G. Abellan, et al., 2006, *Journal of Nutritional Health and Aging, 10,* pp. 456–465. Screening for Undernutrition in Geriatric Practice: Developing the Short-Form Mini Nutritional Assessment (MNA-SF), by L. Z. Rubenstein, J. O. Harker, A. Salva, Y. Guigoz, & B. Vellas, 2001, *Journal of Gerontology, 56A,* pp. M366–M377. The Mini-Nutritional Assessment (MNA®) Review of the Literature: What Does It Tell Us?, by Y. Guigoz, 2006, *Journal of Nutritional Health and Aging, 10,* pp. 466–487. For more information: http://www.mna-elderly.com

5.2 MyPyramid food guide.

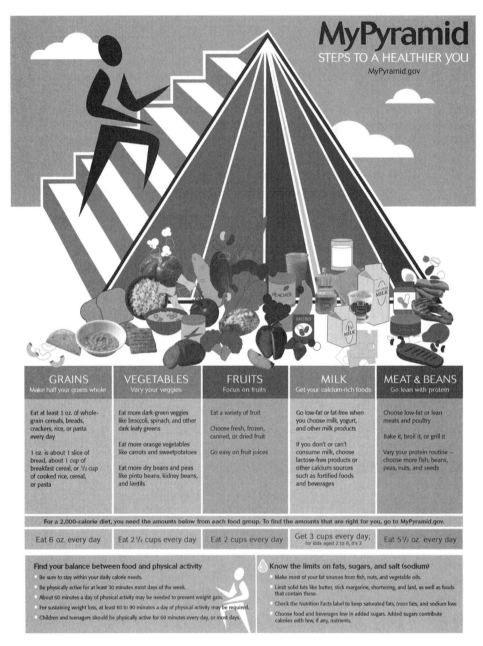

Note. From U.S. Department of Agriculture, Center for Nutrition Policy and Promotion, CNPP=15. (2005, April). Retrieved April 15, 2008, from http://www.MyPyramid.gov

asleep and frequent night-time awakenings. About half of older adults report one or more sleep problems. Key indicators of sleep disorders include

■ Prolonged periods of difficulty falling asleep or getting back to sleep after night-time awakenings
■ Daytime fatigue or sleepiness

Sleep patterns are affected by both normal and pathological aging changes. Sleep assessment is the first key to successful sleep management (see Exhibit 5.1). Sleep interventions include the following:

■ Increase physical activity during the day.
■ Increase pain medication or alternative pain methods to help older adults suffering from painful conditions to get better rest at night.
■ Examine the sleep environment. Adjustments in noise and lighting may help older adults to sleep better.
■ Assess the stress in the lives of older adults. Identification and resolution of stressful life factors may help older adults to sleep more peacefully.
■ Daytime napping tends to interfere with a good night's sleep. Older adults who choose to nap during the day should acknowledge that the napping will likely reduce the total nighttime sleep needed.

Adult Immunization

One of the greatest advances in primary prevention and public health has been the use of immunizations to prevent disease. Adult immunization guidelines are given in Figure 5.3. Two vaccine-preventable diseases that occur commonly in the elderly with great risk for morbidity and mortality are influenza and viral pneumonia. Influenza results in approximately 42.7 million hospitalizations and deaths annually. Despite this high number and the availability of a preventable vaccine, less than 60% of community-dwelling older adults get vaccinated each year.

A major Healthy People 2010 objective is to increase influenza vaccination among all older adults, especially those with:

■ Respiratory disorders
■ Chronic heart diseases
■ Chronic renal disease
■ Immunosuppression

Vaccination is contraindicated in people who are allergic to eggs and in those who have experienced a reaction to the vaccine in the past. Pneumonia is an infectious disease caused by several possible organisms.

■ Pneumonia is the leading cause of death from infectious disease in the United States.
■ It is the sixth leading cause of death overall.

5.3 Recommended adult immunization schedule, United States, 2003–2004.

by Age Group

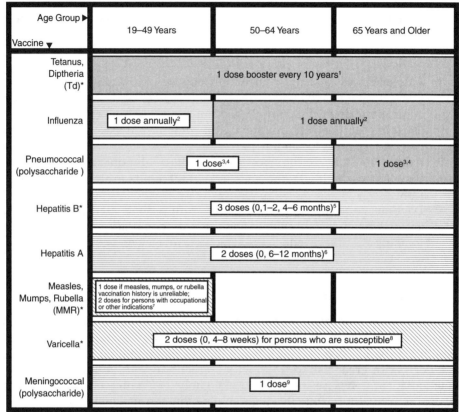

Age Group ▶ Vaccine ▼	19–49 Years	50–64 Years	65 Years and Older
Tetanus, Diptheria (Td)*	1 dose booster every 10 years[1]		
Influenza	1 dose annually[2]	1 dose annually[2]	
Pneumococcal (polysaccharide)	1 dose[3,4]		1 dose[3,4]
Hepatitis B*	3 doses (0,1–2, 4–6 months)[5]		
Hepatitis A	2 doses (0, 6–12 months)[6]		
Measles, Mumps, Rubella (MMR)*	1 dose if measles, mumps, or rubella vaccination history is unreliable; 2 doses for persons with occupational or other indications[7]		
Varicella*	2 doses (0, 4–8 weeks) for persons who are susceptible[8]		
Meningococcal (polysaccharide)	1 dose[9]		

See Footnotes for Recommended Adult Immunization Schedule, by Age Group and Medical Conditions, United States, 2003–2004 on back cover

▓ For all persons in this group   ╲ Catch-up on childhood vaccinations   ≡ For persons with medical/ exposure indications

* Covered by the Vaccine Injury Compensation Program. For information on how to file a claim call 800-338-2382. Please also visit www.hrsa.gov/osp/vicp To file a claim for vaccine injury contact: U.S. Court of Federal Claims, 717 Madison Place, N.W., Washington D.C. 20005, 202-2199657

This schedule indicates the recommended age groups for routine administration of currently licensed vaccines for persons 19 years of age and older. Licensed combination vaccines may be used whenever any components of the combination are indicated and the vaccine's other components are not contraindicated. Providers should consult the manufacturers' package inserts for detailed recommendations.

Report all clinically significant post-vaccination reactions to the Vaccine Adverse Event Reporting System (VAERS). Reporting forms and instructions on filing a VAERS report are available by calling 800-822-7967 or from the VAERS website at http://vaers.hhs.gov/ .

For additional information about the vaccines listed above and contraindications for immunization, visit the National Immunization Program Website at www.cdc.gov/nip or call the National Immunization Hotline at 800-232-2522 (English) or 800-232-0233 (Spanish).

Approved by the Advisory Committee on Immunization Practices (ACIP), and accepted by the American College of Obstetricians and Gynecologists (ACOG) and the American Academy of Family Physicians (AAFP)

by Medical Conditions

Medical Conditions ▼ / Vaccine ▶	Tetanus-Diphtheria (Td)*,1	Influenza[2]	Pneumococcal (polysaccharide)[3,4]	Hepatitis B*,[5]	Hepatitis A[6]	Measles, Mumps, Rubella (MMR)*,[7]	Varicella*,[8]
Pregnancy		A					
Diabetes, heart disease, chronic pulmonary disease, chronic liver disease, including chronic alcoholism		B	C		D		
Congenital Immunodeficiency, leukemia, lymphoma, generalized malignancy, therapy with alkylating agents, antimetabolites, radiation or large amounts of corticosteroids			E				F
Renal failure / end stage renal disease, recipients of hemodialysis or clotting factor concentrates			E	G			
Asplenia including elective splenectomy and terminal complement component deficiencies		H	E, I, J				
HIV infection			E, K			L	

See Special Notes for Medical Conditions below—also see Footnotes for Recommended Adult Immunization Schedule, by Age Group and Medical Conditions, United States, 2003–2004 on back cover

- ▨ For all persons in this group
- ▨ Catch-up on childhood vaccinations
- ≡ For persons with medical / exposure indications
- ■ Contraindicated

Special Notes for Medical Conditions

A. For women without chronic diseases/conditions, vaccinate if pregnancy will be at 2nd or 3rd trimester during influenza season. For women with chronic diseases/conditions, vaccinate at any time during pregnancy.

B. Although chronic liver disease and alcoholism are not indicator conditions for influenza vaccination, give 1 dose annually if the patient is age 50 years or older, has other indications for influenza vaccine, or if the patient requests vaccination.

C. Asthma is an indicator condition for influenza but not for pneumococcal vaccination.

D. For all persons with chronic liver disease.

E. For persons < 65 years, revaccinate once after 5 years or more have elapsed since initial vaccination.

F. Persons with impaired humoral immunity but intact cellular immunity may be vaccinated. *MMWR* 1999; 48 (RR-06):1-5

G. Hemodialysis patients: Use special formulation of vaccine (40 ug/mL) or two 1.0 mL 20 ug doses given at one site. Vaccinate early in the course of renal disease. Assess antibody titers to hep B surface antigen (anti-HBs) levels annually. Administer additional doses if anti-HBs levels decline to <10 milliinternational units (mIU)/mL.

H. There are no data specifically on risk of severe or complicated influenza infections among persons with asplenia. However, influenza is a risk factor for secondary bacterial infections that may cause severe disease in asplenics.

I. Administer meningococcal vaccine and consider Hib vaccine.

J. Elective splenectomy: vaccinate at least 2 weeks before surgery.

K. Vaccinate as close to diagnosis as possible when CD4 cell counts are highest.

L. Withhold MMR or other measles containing vaccines from HIV-infected persons with evidence of severe immunosuppression. *MMWR* 1998; 47 (RR-8):21–22; *MMWR* 2002; 51 (RR-02):22–24.

5.1 The Pittsburgh Sleep Quality Index (PSQI)

Instructions: The following questions relate to your usual sleep habits during the past month only. Your answers should indicate the most accurate reply for the majority of days and nights in the past month. Please answer all questions.
During the past month,
1. When have you usually gone to bed? _____
2. How long (in minutes) has it taken you to fall asleep each night? _____
3. When have you usually gotten up in the morning? _____
4. How many hours of actual sleep do you get at night? (This may be different than the number of hours you spend in bed.) _____

5. During the past month, how often have you had trouble sleeping because you…	Not during the past month (0)	Less than once a week (1)	Once or twice a week (2)	Three or more times a week (3)
a. Cannot get to sleep within 30 minutes				
b. Wake up in the middle of the night or early morning				
c. Have to get up to use the bathroom				
d. Cannot breathe comfortably				
e. Cough or snore loudly				
f. Feel too cold				
g. Feel too hot				
h. Have bad dreams				
i. Have pain				
j. Other reason(s), please describe, including how often you have had trouble sleeping because of this reason(s):				
6. During the past month, how often have you taken medicine (prescribed or over the counter) to help you sleep?				
7. During the past month, how often have you had trouble staying awake while driving, eating meals, or engaging in social activity?				
8. During the past month, how much of a problem has it been for you to keep up enthusiasm to get things done?				
	Very good (0)	Fairly good (1)	Fairly bad (2)	Very bad (3)
9. During the past month, how would you rate your sleep quality overall?				

Component 1   #9 Score ....C1_____
Component 2   #2 Score (≤ 15 min = 0; 16–30 min = 1; 31–60 min =2, > 60 min = 3) + #5a Score
                (if sum is equal 0 = 0; 1–2 = 1; 3–4 = 2; 5–6 = 3) ....C2_____
Component 3   #4 Score (> 7 = 0; 6–7 = 1; 5–6 = 2; <5 = 3) ....C3_____
Component 4   (total # of hours asleep)/(total # of hours in bed) x 100
                > 85% = 0, 75%–84% = 1, 65%–74% = 2, < 65% = 3 ....C4_____
Component 5   Sum of Scores #5b to #5j (0 = 0; 1–9 = 1; 10–18 = 2; 19–27 = 3) ....C5_____
Component 6   #6 Score ....C6_____
Component 7   #7 Score + #8 Score (0 = 0; 1–2 = 1; 3-4 = 2; 5–6 = 3)..............................C7_____

                    Add the seven component scores together _____ **Global PSQI Score** _____

Note. Reprinted from "The Pittsburgh Sleep Quality Index: A New Instrument for Psychiatric Practice and Research," by D. J. Buysse, C. F. Reynolds III, T. H. Monk, S. R. Berman, and D. J. Kupfer, 1989, *Journal of Psychiatric Research, 28* (2), pp. 193–213. Copyright 1989, with permission from Elsevier Science.

- Estimates indicate that pneumococcal infections are responsible for approximately 100,000 deaths per year.
- Pneumonia vaccination is recommended every 10 years or more frequently in high-risk populations.
- Many older adults are unvaccinated against pneumonia.
- Pneumonia vaccine is effective at preventing 56% to 81% of viral infections.
- Pneumonia vaccine is estimated to prevent 80% of pneumonia-related deaths.
- The vaccine is not useful in some immunocompromised patients.
- Indications for the pneumonia vaccine:

  - Everyone older than 65 years
  - People ages 2 to 64 who have chronic illness or live in high-risk areas
  - Older adults with chronic lung, heart, kidney, sickle cell disease, or diabetes

Alternative and Complementary Health Care

The use of herbal medications to treat commonly occurring normal and pathological changes of aging has grown considerably over the past decade. The Gerontological Society of America (2004) reports that one-third of older adults used alternative medicine in 2002.

Herbal medications may be preferred over traditional medication among many cultural groups including Chinese and other Asian cultures. The availability of these herbals, often referred to as nutraceuticals, and the anecdotal evidence of their effectiveness have spawned the sudden growth in sales of these supplements. Nutraceuticals also tend to be less expensive than prescription drugs.

The Gerontological Society of America (2004) reports that their perceived effectiveness and lower cost led to 13% of older adults turning to herbal medications over prescriptions to treat medical problems.

Herbal supplements commonly used by older adults:

- Vitamins C, D, and E, which have shown some evidence of reducing symptoms of osteoarthritis. However, vitamin E has been shown to result in increased risk of bleeding disorders.
- Ginger and glucosamine have also been used extensively by older adults to reduce arthritis-related pain. However, glucosamine may interfere with insulin and oral hypoglycemic medications in diabetic patients.
- Black licorice has been thought to reduce joint inflammation to reduce symptoms of arthritis but may cause irregular heart rhythms and may interact with some diuretics and vitamin K.
- Gingko biloba is widely used by older adults to enhance memory, but it has been shown to increase the risk of bleeding disorders.
- Saw palmetto is used by many older men to reduce symptoms of enlarged prostate glands and to prevent prostate cancer. However, this

nutraceutical may falsely lower prostate specific antigen levels and has been shown to result in increased risk of bleeding disorders.
▧ Ginseng is used by older adults to reduce stress.
▧ St. John's wort is often used as an alternative or adjunct treatment for depression.
▧ Cascara sagrada may result in hypokalemia.

A summary of commonly used herbal medications and their indications is provided in Table 5.2.

5.2	Herbal Components Under Study by the National Toxicology Program
Aloe vera gel	Widely used herb, both as a dietary supplement and component of cosmetics. Ninth highest in sales in the United States (2002). The gel has been used for centuries as a treatment for minor burns and is increasingly being used in products for internal consumption.
Black cohosh	Used to treat symptoms of premenstrual syndrome, dysmenorrhea, and menopause. Ranked 11th in sales in 2002.
Bladderwrack	A source of iodide used in treatment of thyroid diseases and also used as a component of weight-loss preparations.
Comfrey	Herb consumed in teas and as fresh leaves for salads; however, it contains pyrrolizidine alkaloids (e.g., symphatine), which are known to be toxic. Used externally as an anti-inflammatory agent in the treatment of bruises, sprains, and other external wounds. Based in part on NTP studies on the alkaloid components of comfrey, the FDA has recommended that manufacturers of dietary supplements containing this herb remove them from the market.
Echinacea pur-purea extract	The most commonly used medicinal herb in the United States (2002). Used as an immunostimulant to treat colds, sore throat, and flu.
Ephedra	Also known as Ma Huang; 21st in sales in 2002. Traditionally used as a treatment for symptoms of asthma and upper respiratory infections. Often found in weight loss and "energy" preparations, which usually also contain caffeine. Use has been associated with side effects such as heart palpitations, psychiatric and upper gastrointestinal effects, and symptoms of autonomic hyperactivity such as tremor and insomnia, especially when taken with other stimulants.
Ginkgo biloba extract	Fourth highest in sales (2002). Ginkgo fruit and seeds have been used medicinally for thousands of years. The extract of green-picked leaves has shown increasing popularity in the United States. Ginkgo biloba extract promotes vasodilatation and improved blood flow and appears beneficial, particularly for short-term memory loss, headache, and depression.

(continued)

5.2 Herbal Components Under Study by the National Toxicology Program (*continued*)

Ginseng and ginsenosides	Ginseng ranked 13th in sales of medicinal herbs in 2002 down from 4th in 1996. Ginsenosides are thought to be the active ingredients. Ginseng has been used as a treatment for a variety of conditions including hypertension, diabetes, and depression, and been associated with various adverse health effects.
Goldenseal	Seventeenth in sales (2002). Traditionally used to treat wounds, digestive problems, and infections. Current uses include as a laxative, tonic, and diuretic. Mistakenly thought to disguise the presence of other drugs in drug tests.
Green tea extract	Used for its antioxidative properties, 15th in sales in 2002.
Kava kava	The 25th most widely used medicinal herb (2002), kava kava has psychoactive properties and is sold as a calmative and antidepressant. A recent report of severe liver toxicity has led to restrictions of its sale in Europe and has apparently affected sales in the United States. Some components may alter efficacy/toxicity of therapeutic agents.
Milk thistle extract	Ranked eighth in sales in 2002. Used to treat depression and several liver conditions including cirrhosis and hepatitis and to increase breast milk production.
Pulegone	A major terpenoid constituent of the herb, Pennyroyal, is found in lesser concentrations in other mints. Pennyroyal has been used as a carminative insect repellent, emmenagogue, and abortifacient. Pulegone has well-recognized toxicity to the liver, kidney, and central nervous system.
Senna	Laxative with increased use due to the removal of one of the widely used chemical-stimulant type laxatives from the market. Study in p53+/− transgenic mice is in progress.
Thujone	Terpenoid found in a variety of herbs, including sage and tansy, and in high concentrations in wormwood. Suspected as the causative toxic agent associated with drinking absinthe, a liqueur flavored with wormwood extract.

Note. From National Toxicology Program. Medicinal herbs. Retrieved March 23, 2008, from http://ntp.niehs.nih.gov/files/herbalfacts06.pdf

References

Buysse, D. J., Reynolds III, C. F., Monk, T. H., Berman, S. R., & Kupfer, D. J. (1989). The Pittsburgh Sleep Quality Index: A new instrument for psychiatric practice and research. *Journal of Psychiatric Research, 28*(2), 193–213.

Centers for Disease Control and Merck Institute for Aging and Health. (2004). The state of aging and health in America. Retrieved July 13, 2007, from http://www.cdc.gov/aging/pdf/State_of_Aging_and_Health_in_America_2004.pdf

Gerontological Society of America. (2004, July). Alternative medicine gains popularity. *Gerontology News, 4,* 3.

Guigoz, Y. (2006). The mini-nutritional assessment (MNA®) review of the literature: What does it tell us? *Journal of Nutritional Health and Aging, 10,* 466–487.

Lichtenstein, A. H., Rasmussen, H., Yu, W. W., Epstein, S. R., & Russell, R. M. (2008). Modified MyPyramid for older adults. *Journal of Nutrition Commentary,* 5–11.

National Toxicology Program. (2008). Medicinal herbs. Retrieved March 23, 2008, from http://ntp.niehs.nih.gov/files/herbalfacts06.pdf

Rubenstein, L. Z., Harker, J. O., Salva, A., Guigoz, Y., & Vellas, B. (2001). Screening for undernutrition in geriatric practice: Developing the short-form mini nutritional assessment (MNA-SF). *Journal of Gerontology, 56A,* M366–M377.

Vellas, B., Villars, H., Abellan, G., et al. (2006). Overview of the MNA®: Its history and challenges. *Journal of Nutritional Health and Aging, 10,* 456–465.

6

Environments of Care

Safety and Security Issues

Falls

Preventing falls and traumas is an important issue for nurses caring for older adults. Falls among older adults in every care setting are a large national problem. Approximately one-third of older adults living at home and up to two-thirds of older adults in long-term care facilities fall each year. When an older adult falls, the consequences may be devastating.

- They are likely to develop a fracture.
- This may begin a spiral of iatrogenesis.
- The result may be death.

The National Center for Health Statistics annual mortality report shows that fall-related deaths among older adults increased sharply between 1998 and 2006. Older men tend to die from falls; older women experience more hospitalizations for fall-related hip fracture. Normal changes of aging contribute to falls, including

- Sensory alterations
- Visual and hearing declines
- Changes in urinary function

Pathological aging changes also contribute to falls, including

- Cognitive disorders
- Osteoporosis
- Strokes
- Sensory impairments

The highest risk factor for an older adult having a fall is a history of a previous fall.

- Fall prevention is critical to preventing the negative consequences of falling among older adults.
- Prevention begins with assessment (see Table 6.1).
- Prevention strategies include

  - Removal of fall hazards such as area rugs
  - Appropriate nonglaring lighting
  - Wall-to-wall carpeting or padding on the floor next to the bed
  - Bed and chair alarms to alert caregivers of older adult mobility

Use of Restraints

Despite the high risk and negative consequences of falls among older adults, restraints are not a reasonable fall prevention intervention. A physical restraint is defined as a device or object attached or adjacent to a person's body that cannot be removed easily and restricts freedom of movement. Several types of restraints are available.

- Physical restraints

  - Side rails on hospital beds
  - Jackets
  - Belts
  - Wrist restraints

- Chemical restraints

  - Sedatives
  - Hypnotics

Evidence about the negative effects of the use of restraints is so disturbing that the mandate for restraint-free care can no longer be ignored. Significant morbidity and mortality risk—including asphyxiation and strangulation—is associated with the use of physical restraints, especially when patients are

- Confused
- Agitated

6.1 Hendrich II Fall Risk Model™

Confusion Disorientation Impulsivity	4	
Symptomatic Depression	2	
Altered Elimination	1	
Dizziness Vertigo	1	
Male Gender	1	
Any Administered Antiepileptics	2	
Any Administered Benzodiazepines	1	
Get Up & Go Test		
Able to rise in a single movement–No Loss of Balance with Steps	0	
Pushes up, successful in one attempt	1	
Multiple attempts, but successful	3	
Unable to rise without assistance during test (OR if a medical order states the same and/or complete bed rest is ordered) *If unable to assess, document this on the patient chart with the date and time	4	
A Score of 5 or Greater = High Risk Total Score		

Note. Copyright © 2007 AHI of Indiana Inc. All rights reserved. United States Patent £7,282,031. Federal Laws prohibits the replication, distribution or use without written permission from AHI of Indiana Incorporated

■ Experiencing new onset pressure ulcer
■ Suffering from pneumonia
■ Neurologically impaired

Older adults should only be restrained if they are in immediate, physical danger or are hurting themselves or others and then for only a brief period of time. The Omnibus Budget Reconciliation Act of 1987 attempted to curtail restraint use in long-term care facilities. Restraint alternatives should be implemented to keep residents safe from falls.

■ Wall-to-wall carpeting
■ Mattress placed on the floor
■ Personal attendants
■ Chair or bed alarms

Hypo- and Hyperthermia

Due to normal and pathological aging, including reduction in the number of pyrogenes, older adults tend to have difficulty regulating heat and cold. Many older adults die each year from hyperthermia-related heat stroke in the summer due to exposure to extreme temperatures and inability to regulate heat though sweating. Heat stroke is the most serious form of hyperthermia and may result in death if not treated immediately. Many older adults also die each year from hypothermia, which could be reduced through exercise among older adults.

Relocation

Older adults reside in a variety of care environments:

- Home
- Senior housing
- Nursing home
- Assisted living
- Continuing care retirement communities
- The street

Relocation is a significant life event that may play a role in the development or severity of depression among older adults. Relocation of older adults occurs commonly as a result of

- Illness
- Decline in functional status
- Loss of spouse or significant other
- Changes in economic status caused by retirement or the death of the family provider

Because of the negative consequences of relocation, *aging in place* is emphasized as a concept that refers to remaining in one setting throughout the majority of older adulthood.

Translocation syndrome results from a change in surroundings from a home to a nursing home or assisted living facility and may trigger the onset of delirium. The syndrome may manifest as

- Impaired physical health
- Depression
- Disruption of established behavior patterns
- Disruption of social relationships

Translocation from one environment to another may potentially upset the patient. Attempting to transition the patient smoothly to his or her new environment is important.

- Letting older adults bring favorite things to their new environment helps them transition more effectively.

■ Empowering older adults as much as possible by allowing them to make decisions and articulate needs and desires is a critical factor in assisting their adjustment from one environment to another.

■ One intervention is to orient the patient regularly and to reassure his or her safety.

Translocation syndrome is likely to happen during admission to a nursing home or transfer to acute care from a nursing home environment.

■ Close attention to the transition of an older adult across environments of care is essential to minimize the symptoms of translocation syndrome.

■ Older adults must continually be assessed for alterations in function and cognition and be supported to participate in the environment at the highest possible level.

■ Changes in function, cognition, and affect must be diagnosed immediately and appropriate interventions implemented to ensure as safe a transition as possible.

■ Little research is available regarding relocation stress and translocation of older adults.

Transportation

Many older adults continue to drive. As the percentage of older adults living in the United States continues to increase, the number of older drivers will also rise. The risk for injuries, hospitalizations, and death from automobile accidents is increased in the older adult population because of the many normal and pathological changes in the neuromuscular and sensory systems, listed in Table 6.2. The number of elderly traffic fatalities is expected to more than triple by the year 2030, exceeding the number of alcohol-related fatalities in 1995 by 35% (Burkhardt, Berger, Creedon, & McGavock, 1998).

The growth in the number of older drivers presents additional problems, because cars, roads, and highways were not developed to accommodate normal changes of aging among older drivers. A large number of older adults thus are unable to safely drive. Driving presents a significant ethical issue of independence among older adults that should not be taken lightly. Older adults who no longer drive face significant issues with transportation. Older adults need transportation for

■ Health care appointments
■ Shopping for food and essentials
■ Socialization

Although van services are available in many communities to transport older adults, they are not universally available.

■ Car and van services usually require advanced scheduling on a first-come, first-served basis.

■ Older adults sometimes have to wait for a long time at a health care facility or physician's office for the van to return to bring them home, extending a short appointment to a day-long outing.

6.2 Normal Aging Changes That Impact Driving

System	Normal aging changes
Sensory	**Vision** ■ Decline in visual acuity ■ Decrease in pupils' ability to constrict in response to stimuli ■ Decline in peripheral vision ■ Yellowing of the lens **Hearing** ■ Increased prevalence of hearing disorders
Neurological	■ Slower response time to stimuli ■ Shift in the proportion of gray matter to white matter ■ Loss of neurons ■ Increase in the number of senile plaques ■ Decreased blood flow to the cerebrum

■ Public transportation such as buses or subway systems may be used by older adults to attend their medical appointments.
■ Public transportation systems have increased accessibility to accommodate disabilities among older adults.
■ Long walks to bus or subway stations may be barriers to public transportation system utilization among the elderly.
■ Caregivers, friends, and neighbors are often relied upon for transportation among older adults.
■ The barriers presented by transportation to health care facilities often force older adults to delay medical treatment for health-related issues.
■ Lack of transportation to purchase food may contribute to malnutrition among older adults.

Territoriality and Personal Space

Most older adults prefer to stay in their own home rather than move to other care environments. Approximately 94% of older adults live in community households, either alone or with a relative. Of the 94% that live in the community, most live alone or with a spouse. Living in the same home environment through life has advantages and disadvantages. Some of the advantages are

■ Ownership and control of one's space and territory
■ The ability to remain among neighbors who share memories and now watch out for each other
■ The opportunity to function as parents or grandparents to new families who move into the neighborhood

Some of the disadvantages of remaining at home:

- Many homes require costly and difficult repairs and maintenance that some older adults can no longer afford or manage.
- Decline in functional status, vision, and hearing can make adaptation to a home and socialization difficult.
- Medical care and assistance with activities of daily living and instrumental activities of daily living are not built into the home.
- Older adults typically have to leave home to obtain care or hire outside providers.
- The latter may be costly, and expenses are not always covered by Medicare and private insurance.
- Although they may not be reimbursable, many health care services are available in the home, including
  - Nursing
  - Physical therapy
  - Occupational therapy
  - Speech-language pathology
  - Assistance with personal care
  - Social work

If an older adult can no longer live at home, attention should be given to protection of his or her territory and personal space in alternate care settings. Territoriality involves setting boundaries to protect one's personal space. Nurses may help older adults protect their territoriality by

- Suggesting they bring personal items to the new space
- Preventing other staff and residents from invading personal space or crossing boundaries
- Encouraging time in personal space
- Assessing the amount of personal space, the comfort with eye contact, and the use of physical gestures such as hand-shaking to determine the older adult's comfort with these common social norms

Community-Based Services and Resources

Generally, older adults are formally assessed by an agency to determine their need for home care services. Medicare uses the OASIS (outcome and assessment information set) to evaluate possible recipients of home care services. OASIS is a set of data elements that forms a comprehensive assessment for an adult home care patient and provides the basis for measuring patient outcomes for purposes of outcome-based quality improvement. Other community resources funded through grants distributed through Area Agencies on Aging or the federal government include

- Employment resources
- Senior center programs

- Senior housing
- Adult day care services
- Alternative community-based living facilities

It is estimated that family members provide approximately 80% of the care for older adults. Caregiving places a tremendous burden on the caregiver that may result in

- Depression
- Grief
- Fatigue
- Decreased socialization
- Health problems

Respite care for older adults may be found in a local skilled nursing facility so that the caregiver may vacation and rest. Other supportive services may help to ease caregiver burden, such as

- Home health aides
- Homemakers
- Chore services
- Meals on Wheels

Caregivers must be encouraged and supported to take care of themselves and pursue their own interests and activities.

Residential Facilities

Several types of residential facilities perform care for older adults.

Skilled Nursing Facilities

Skilled nursing facilities (SNFs) may be private or public and may receive reimbursement from Medicare, Medicaid, and private insurances, or residents may self-pay.

- Nursing services provided in SNFs may include
    - Medication administration
    - Wound care
    - Daily assessment
    - Meals
    - Assistance with activities of daily living
    - Physical therapy
    - Respiratory therapy
    - Speech-language pathology services
    - Occupational therapy

■ Short-term rehabilitation after surgery or medical illness
■ Lifetime residential services

The documentation specific to skilled nursing facilities is known as the Minimum Data Set (MDS). This is a core set of screening, clinical, and functional status elements, including common definitions and coding categories.

■ The MDS is the foundation of the comprehensive assessment for all residents of long-term care facilities certified to participate in Medicare or Medicaid.
■ The MDS standardizes communication about resident problems and conditions within facilities, between facilities, and between facilities and outside agencies.

Assisted Living Facilities

Assisted living facilities (ALFs) were developed in the 1980s to provide supportive residential housing for the rapidly growing elderly population. ALFs place a greater emphasis on autonomy. They are appealing housing alternatives to older adults with minor to moderate functional impairments. ALFs generally follow a nonmedical, homelike model, focusing on resident

■ Autonomy
■ Privacy
■ Independence
■ Dignity
■ Respect

ALFs are less expensive than SNFs, but the nonmedical model also precludes reimbursement by Medicare. Medicare reimbursement for home care services may be provided by an outside home care agency. Services offered at ALFs vary, but often include

■ 24-hour supervision
■ Three meals a day plus snacks in a dining room setting
■ A range of personal, health care, and recreational services

Services may be included in the monthly rate, or they may be offered at additional costs. Health care and nursing services available at ALFs vary widely throughout the country. Some facilities have adequate 24-hour coverage, while others do not have registered nurses on site. Disparities in state regulations have led to varied interpretations of what ALFs are and what they can do.

Continuing Care Retirement Communities

Continuing care retirement communities (CCRCs) are defined as "full service communities offering long-term contracts that provide for a continuum of care, including retirement, assisted living and nursing services, all on one campus" (New Life Styles, 2005). They are a housing alternative for older adults that arose in the 1980s with the purpose of facilitating aging in place. CCRCs provide several levels of care, including

- Independent living
- Assisted living
- Skilled nursing care

Older adults may remain in the community by changing the level of care they receive as changes occur in their health, functional, or cognitive status. CCRCs are very expensive and require an entrance fee and a monthly payment. However,

- Skilled levels of care are reimbursable under Medicare.
- Independent and assisted living are privately paid.
- Periodic home care services may be reimbursable under Medicare by home care nurses.

Residence in a CCRC requires a commitment to a long-term contract that specifies the housing, services, and nursing care provided. AARP (2007) reports that there are three types of CCRC contracts:

- Extensive contracts include unlimited long-term nursing care at minimal or no increase in monthly fee.
- Modified contracts include a specified amount of long-term care. If chronic conditions require more care beyond the specified time, the older adult is responsible for payments.
- With fee-for-service contracts, the older adult pays the full daily rates for long-term nursing care.

CCRCs originated from religious or social groups interested in caring for members of their communities. More recently, private investors have begun to purchase and operate these communities. Services provided depend on the level of care and range from

- Basic recreational services in independent living to
- Full care and meals in a skilled nursing environment

Homeless Elders

Homelessness is a significant problem among the older adult population. Little is known about the homeless older population because they rarely seek health services, and thus they are difficult to access. The few available studies estimate that there are between 60,000 and 400,000 older homeless adults in the United States. The typical older homeless person is a man. Despite the lack of health service use among older homeless adults, this population suffers from

- Substantial physical disease
- Mental illness
- Alcohol abuse
- Drug abuse

These risk factors increase the prevalence of the following conditions among homeless older adults:

- Morbidity
- Mortality
- Decreased bone density
- Malnutrition
- Hip fracture from falls
- Motor vehicle accidents

References

American Association of Retired Persons (AARP). (2007). Continuing care retirement communities. Retrieved July 14, 2007, from http://www.aarp.org/families/housing_choices/other_options/a2004-02-26-retirementcommunity.html

Burkhardt, J. E., Berger, A. M., Creedon, M., & McGavock, A. T. (1998). *Mobility and independence: Changes and challenges for older drivers.* Washington, DC: Department of Health and Human Services (DHHS), under the auspices of the Joint DHHS/DOT Coordinating Council on Access and Mobility.

New Life Styles. (2005). Types of senior housing and care. Retrieved August 25, 2007, from http://www.newlifestyles.com/resources/articles/Selecting_a_Continuing.aspx

Spirituality and Death and Dying

Dying is a natural last stage of life. As people approach the end of life, they may explore the meaning of life and question the possibility of an afterlife. Just because older adults are closer to a natural death than young people, they are not necessarily prepared to die. The many aspects of end-of-life nursing care include

- Communication
- Physical care
- Spiritual care
- Emotional care
- Psychological care
- Assistance with family grieving

Principles of Effective End-of-Life Care

The goal of end-of-life nursing care is to help patients experience a "good death." Palliative care is aimed at providing essential elements to ensure a good death.

The World Health Organization (2005) defines palliative care as "the active total care of patients whose disease is not responsive to curative treatment. Control of pain, other symptoms, and psychological, social, and spiritual problems is paramount."

The four dimensions of end-of-life care are physical, psychological, social, and spiritual.

Physical Dimension

The physical dimension of end-of-life care ensures that patients are pain free—no older adult should ever die in pain. Caregivers should follow these guidelines:

- Assess regularly for the presence of pain.
- Treat with pharmacological and nonpharmacological interventions on a regular schedule (not as needed) to ensure the patient is pain free.
- Encourage older adults to maintain their independence as long as possible.
- Assess every day older adults' ability to perform activities of daily living.
- Assistance may be needed when the older adult is no longer able to complete activities of daily living independently.
- Other physical symptoms common at the end of life include dyspnea, cough, anorexia, constipation, diarrhea, nausea, vomiting, and fatigue. These symptoms are summarized in Table 7.1.

Psychological Dimension

The psychological dimension of end-of-life care focuses on how older adults feel about themselves and their relationships with others. Are there unresolved personal issues? Are there unfinished tasks that need to be completed so that the older adult can feel that his or her responsibilities have been met?

- The older adult's success in meeting the developmental tasks of aging must be assessed.
- The end of life provides an opportunity to complete important developmental tasks of aging.
- Discussing issues with older adults who are approaching the end of life will help to identify uncompleted tasks.
- Although it may seem too late, some older adults have
  - Completed academic degrees
  - Contacted estranged family members
  - Been married on their death beds
- The nurse may be the one to make the phone call or mediate the discussion between two people who have not spoken in years.

7.1 Physical Symptoms at the End of Life

Physical symptom	Nursing interventions
Dyspnea	▪ Assess respiratory rate and effort as well as pattern of dyspnea and triggering and relieving factors (i.e., activity).
	▪ Respiratory rates of more than 20 breaths per minute, labored respirations, use of accessory muscles, and diminished or adventitious lung sounds require follow-up and possible intervention.
	▪ Administer morphine solution orally, sublingually, or via suppository every 2 hours as needed. Diuretics (e.g., Lasix), bronchodilators, steroids, antibiotics, anticholinergics, and sedatives should also be considered.
	▪ Administer oxygen as appropriate to relieve symptoms, especially in those who do not respond to morphine.
	▪ Keep environment cool and position client for full chest expansion.
Cough	▪ Assess etiology of cough.
	▪ If from excess fluids, treat accordingly with diuretics (e.g., Lasix).
	▪ Reduce smoking and make sure environmental air is clear, cool, and humidified.
	▪ Elevate head of bed.
	▪ Ensure proper fluid administration.
	▪ Administer cough suppressants/depressants, opiates, bronchodilators, and local anesthetics.
Anorexia	▪ Understand that lack of hunger is normal at the end of life. Food and fluids at the end of life may create distress and, thus, anorexia does not necessarily need to be treated.
	▪ Good mouth care, using a soft toothbrush or spongy oral swab, is essential to prevent dryness, mouth sores, dental problems, and infections.
	▪ If the client can tolerate fluids, provide soups, tomato juice, and sport drinks to prevent electrolyte imbalances.
Constipation	▪ Recognize the impact of morphine preparations on constipation among older adults and administer prophylactic treatment for constipation.
	▪ Assess client's self-report as well as physical symptoms of constipation such as bowel distension, nausea, vomiting, or rectal impaction.
	▪ Recommended medications include stool softeners such as docusate sodium (Colace) and stimulant laxatives such as senna (Sennakot-S).

(continued)

7.1 Physical Symptoms at the End of Life (*continued*)

Physical symptom	Nursing interventions
	▪ Bowel suppositories and enemas may also be used to relieve constipation.
	▪ Be alert for the progression of constipation to bowel obstruction. This may present as steady abdominal pain and is a medical emergency.
Diarrhea	▪ Assess presence and etiology of diarrhea and remove cause, if possible.
	▪ Ensure adequate fiber and bulk in diet and adequate fluids.
	▪ Determine times throughout the day when older adults are most often incontinent through a bowel diary.
	▪ Once the pattern of incontinent episodes is determined, the older adult may be encouraged and assisted to the toilet a half-hour before diarrhea usually occurs.
	▪ Consider the administration of diphenoxylate (Lomotil) or loperamide (Imodium).
Nausea and vomiting	▪ Assess client's self-report of nausea, along with aggravating and relieving factors. The use of a diary may be helpful.
	▪ Assess vomiting as well as aggravating and relieving factors. It is important to note that retching and gagging may occur even in unresponsive clients.
	▪ Administer antiemetics around the clock (not as needed). Antiemetics that may be effective include prochlorperazine (Compazine) and metoclopramide (Reglan) administered as a rectal suppository, intravenously, or parenterally.
	▪ Consider the combination preparation of lorazepam (Ativan), diphenhydramine (Benadryl), haloperidol (Haldol), and metochlopramide (Reglan) if antiemetics alone are not effective at relieving symptoms.
Fatigue	▪ Fatigue must be recognized as a major source of distress among older adults at the end of life and has a great impact on quality of life.
	▪ Treatment of symptoms such as pain, nausea, vomiting, and dyspnea significantly impact fatigue.
	▪ Light exercise and activity alternating with periods of rest and relaxation are effective at relieving fatigue.
	▪ Music and guided imagery may also be helpful for inducing rest and providing stimulation during fatigued periods.

Note. Adapted from *Palliative Care Nursing: Quality of Care to the End of Life,* by M. L. Matzo and D. W. Sherman (Eds.), 2006, New York: Springer Publishing.

- Nurses can play an important role in helping older adults to complete these developmental tasks and experience a good death.
- The end of life often involves the development of depression, anxiety, confusion, agitation, and delirium. These symptoms and suggested nursing interventions are described in Table 7.2.

Social Dimension

The social dimension of end-of-life care identifies roles that older adults have occupied and determines whether they have disengaged from these roles. With the rising number of older adults caring for grandchildren, an aging grandmother may be concerned about who will care for her grandchildren when she passes away.

- Older adults may be employed and worry about how their job responsibilities will be met upon their death.
- Older adults may be caregivers to ill or cognitively impaired spouses or siblings, and the loved one's future care is likely to be a concern.

Spiritual Dimension

The spiritual dimension of end-of-life care allows the older adult to transcend from this life into another existence.

- If the older adult has explored the meaning of his or her life and has an expectation of an afterlife, death may be peaceful.
- Older adults often continue to struggle with the meaning of life even at the end.
- The presence of spirituality in the lives of older adults once was not acknowledged.
- The original work of Rowe and Kahn (1997) on successful aging neglected to include the component of spirituality.
- More recently, spirituality has been identified as an integral component of health and functioning.
- Spirituality provides a framework within which people conduct the search for meaning and purpose in life.
- Spirituality differs from religion, which specifically concerns the spiritual beliefs and practices held by organized groups (e.g., Buddhist, Catholic, Protestant, Jewish).
- Religion is defined by Koenig et al. (2001) as "an organized system of beliefs, practices, rituals and symbols designed
  a. to facilitate closeness to the sacred or transcendent (God, higher power, or ultimate truth/reality)
  b. to foster an understanding of one's relation and responsibility to others living together in a community." (p. 18)
- Although many people pursue spirituality through a specific religion, participation in organized religion is not a prerequisite for spirituality.

7.2 Psychological Symptoms at the End of Life

Psychological symptom	Nursing interventions
Depression	■ Assess cause of depression; consider unrelieved pain and anticipatory grieving. ■ Openly discuss older adult's fears and concerns regarding end of life to assist in the resolution of depression. ■ Refer for counseling. ■ Implement suicide precautions, if necessary. ■ Consider administration of antidepressants, including selective serotonin reuptake inhibitors fluoxetine (Prozac), paroxetine (Paxil), and sertraline (Zoloft); tricyclic antidepressants amitriptyline (Elavil), imipramine (Tofranil), and nortriptyline (Pamelor); monoamine oxidase inhibitors phenelzine (Nardil) and tranylcypromine (Parnate); and the other atypical antidepressants (Desyrel) and bupropion (Buspar).
Anxiety and agitation	■ Assess cause of anxiety and agitation; consider unrelieved pain, urinary retention, constipation, and nausea as sources and treat appropriately. ■ Openly discuss older adults' fears and concerns regarding end of life to assist in the resolution of anxiety-producing issues. ■ Administer anxiolytics such as lorazepam (Ativan), diazepam (Valium), or clonazepam (Klonopin). However, remember that these medications may result in delirium among older adults. ■ If anxiolytic medications fail to relieve anxiety, consider the use of barbiturates such as phenobarbital or neuroleptics such as haloperidol (Haldol).
Delirium and acute confusion	■ Assess delirium using a standardized instrument, such as a confusion assessment method. ■ Delirium is a frequent occurrence at end of life as a result of life-threatening conditions and treatment strategies. ■ Immediate detection and removal of the cause of delirium will enhance the patient's recovery to the quickest extent possible. ■ While the delirium is resolving, it is important to keep the older adult safe through the use of detection systems to alert caregivers of wandering behavior and implementing fall prevention strategies. ■ A calm, soft-spoken approach to care is necessary, and the older adult with delirium should not be forced to participate in caregiving activities that cause anxiety or agitation.

Note. Adapted from *Palliative Care Nursing: Quality of Care to the End of Life,* by M. L. Matzo and D. W. Sherman (Eds.), 2006, New York: Springer Publishing.

- Many older adults do not affiliate with an organized religion, yet possess a deep sense of spirituality.
- The importance of spirituality is more readily acknowledged by society, and expressions of spirituality are increasingly diverse.
- While the role of spirituality is strong throughout life for many adults, its role at the end of life is magnified.
- Older adults may explore the meaning of life and question the existence of an afterlife.
- End-of-life care has recently been the subject of a great deal of research, and the role of nursing to promote spiritual health at the end of life is becoming better articulated.
- It is of great importance that nurses understand that spirituality and the practice of religion vary greatly among older adults.
- The presence of spirituality has been associated with relief from physical, mental, and addictive disorders and with enhanced quality of life and survival.
- The influence of spirituality on the health and functioning of older adults as well as a good death indicates the need to plan care that incorporates spiritual needs.
- Older adults who engage in religious and spiritual practice often cope better psychologically and have better physical health than those who don't (Koenig, 2007).
- The presence of spirituality has been associated with relief from physical, mental, and addictive disorders and enhanced quality of life and survival.
- Understanding the role of spirituality in death is the first step toward spiritual care for older adults.
- Spiritual care for older adults begins with an assessment of

  - The individual's beliefs and practices
  - What spirituality means to the client
  - Whether the client is affiliated with a specific religion and is actively involved
  - Whether spirituality is a source of support and strength
  - Whether the client has any special religious traditions, rituals, or practices he or she likes to follow.

- Many spiritual assessment scales are available, including Stoll's Spiritual Assessment Guide and O'Brien's Spiritual Assessment Scale. These instruments may be helpful in conducting spiritual assessments of older adults.
- From the spiritual assessment, deficits in the older adult's spiritual needs may be found and interventions implemented to help the older adult improve his or her spiritual connectedness.
- Nurses should encourage religious and spiritual beliefs and practices in all environments of care, as allowed by institutional policy.
- It is important for nurses to be aware of the availability of religious personnel within each facility and call on these members of the interdisciplinary team to help older adults whenever necessary.

7.3 Cultural Views of Death			
Native Americans	African Americans	Asian Americans	Latin Americans
Death is viewed in a circular pattern rather than linear.	Memories of poor health care might make some older adults concerned about making end-of-life decisions.	End-of-life care decisions may be made by family members who consider it their role, even if the older adult is competent to make decisions. This may also involve the nondisclosure of terminal illness to protect the older adult. Autopsy and organ donation are not accepted, so as not to disturb the body.	Reluctant to make decisions about end-of-life issues or complete advance directives, as well as endorse the withholding or withdrawal of life-prolonging treatment, use hospice services support physician-assisted death, and organ donation. The well-being of the family may be considered over the well-being of the client.

■ Spiritual counseling and praying with the patient can be great sources of comfort to the patient and his or her family.

■ A hallmark of palliative care is communication between caregivers, families, and patients.
■ Nurses can play an instrumental role in bringing together interdisciplinary teams to plan care for dying older adults.
■ Team conferences should be held regularly to plan care and to assess effectiveness in meeting patients' multidimensional palliative care needs.
■ It is important that both the client and family are encouraged to participate in care planning and evaluation.
■ Different cultures view death differently. Cultural views of death are listed in Table 7.3.

Advanced Directives

Advanced directives allow older adults to participate in and direct health care decisions at the end of life or in the event that they are unable to do so at some time in the future. Advanced directives include the right to accept or refuse medical or surgical treatment.

- In 1990, the Patient Self-Determination Act was created to require every health care institution to maintain specific policies and procedures regarding advanced directives for every adult who receives health care in that institution.
- Every older adult has the right to prepare advanced directives and be informed of the provider's policies that govern the utilization of these rights.
- Failure to comply with the act may result in the facility's loss of Medicare and Medicaid payments.
- Advanced directives provide a way for older adults to make decisions about their lives and health care prior to becoming ill. While it is not required that older adults make these decisions (and many do not), it is required that hospitals provide clients with the option to do so.
- The use of verbal statements, living wills, and durable powers of attorney are all considered legitimate advanced directives for future health care treatment decisions.
- Older adults may be encouraged to complete advanced directives in order to have their wishes followed at the end of life.
- Nurses have a unique opportunity to encourage the development of advanced directives in all environments of care.
- Families' decisions about continuing or removing life-sustaining treatments often conflict with health care providers' recommendations. In these cases, it is most appropriate to determine the client's wishes.
- Cultural values influence the decision to sustain or withhold nutrition and hydration at the end of life.
- Verbal statements regarding potential health care problems and possible treatment decisions may be made by older adults to healthcare providers and trusted friends and family.
- Verbal statements indicate a thoughtful approach to decisions that are consistent with ethical principles and with the older adult's past decisions. They may be used to make health care decisions when the older adult is no longer able to do so.
- If verbal statements are spoken to health care providers, documenting them in the patient record provides the best evidence of the patient's wishes.
- Living wills are a written statement about preferences for life-sustaining treatment.
- Living wills provide older adults with the opportunity to describe any life-sustaining treatment they wish to accept or reject should they experience a terminal condition or a permanent state of unconsciousness and are not able to participate in health care treatment decisions.
- Because living wills are written forms generally filed with the older adult's medical record, their usefulness is dependent on the health care providers ability to implement the older adult's wishes.
- Similar to a power of attorney for financial decisions, older adults may designate a trusted person to make health care decisions on their behalf.
- Durable power of attorney for health care or medical power of attorney extends the power to make health care decisions in the event that the decision-making capacity of the older adult is impaired.

- A durable power of attorney may receive diagnostic information, analyze potential treatment options, act as an advocate for the client, and consent to or refuse care.
- A durable power of attorney is a legal advanced directive that offers greater flexibility than a living will.
- The document is not limited to life-sustaining measures; it may apply to nursing home placement, surgery, or other forms of nonemergency treatment.
- The greatest limitation of the durable power of attorney is the requirement of having a person who is willing to serve in the role substitute decision maker.
- If older adults have outlived all their significant others and do not have anyone to serve as a surrogate decision maker, they may petition for or hire a court-appointed power of attorney in order to benefit from the flexibility offered by a durable power of attorney for health care.
- A will is a written document that provides for the distribution of financial assets upon a person's death.
- Wills are important documents to help older adults determine the disposition of their assets, but they do not generally provide advanced direction regarding health care decisions.

Hospice and Palliative Care

Hospice care at the end of life is an extremely valuable, yet underused, resource. Although hospices have provided compassionate palliative care for terminally ill persons and their families in the United States for over 20 years, many people are still not aware of these services.

- The greatest growth in hospice use over the past decade is among older clients (Hospice Association of America, 2007).
- Hospice is a philosophy of care for dying persons and their families that affirms life and empowers dying persons to live with dignity, alert and pain free.
- It involves families and loved ones in giving care that emphasizes quality of life.
- The hospice team facilitates the establishment of an environment where dying persons and their families have satisfactory psychological and spiritual preparation for death.
- The hospice philosophy supports the belief that dying is a natural extension of the living process.
- The traditional goals of hospice care are to

  - Relieve the pain and suffering of the terminally ill
  - Make possible a good death
  - Help the family
  - Assist in the search for the meaning of life and death

Grieving

Nurses' work with older adults at the end of life does not end when the older client passes away. Sadness is a common symptom of the normal mourning process. Nurses can help families through the grieving process. Grieving begins before the older adult dies and proceeds differently for each family.

Types of grief include acute, anticipatory, and dysfunctional.

- Acute grief occurs in response to feelings of loss.
- Anticipatory grief occurs in anticipation of an impending loss.
- Dysfunctional or complicated grief occurs when the duration of symptomatology is prolonged, resulting in impaired psychosocial functioning.

Kubler-Ross (1964) describes several stages of grieving that must be experienced for successful resolution of the loss. Progression through these stages is unpredictable, but necessary.

- Denial (this isn't happening to me)
- Anger (why is this happening to me?)
- Bargaining (I promise I'll be a better person if . . .)
- Depression (I don't care anymore)
- Acceptance (I'm ready for whatever comes)

Families who have lost an older relative never just "get over it."
Signs that a grieving person is in distress may include

- Weight loss
- Substance abuse
- Depression
- Prolonged sleep disorders
- Physical problems
- Suicidal ideation
- Lack of personal hygiene

A grief assessment helps to determine the type of grief, a family's reactions, the stages and tasks to be completed, and additional factors influencing the grief process.

- Once the nurse gathers information on the family's grief, an active listening approach assists with resolution.
- Utilizing principles of therapeutic communication, nurses identify problems with the grieving process and allow the family to talk through their situation, sharing experiences as appropriate so that the family knows they are not alone.
- Nurses may identify support systems, such as bereavement specialists and support groups.
- The nurse should encourage the family to conduct activities and attend rituals surrounding the older adult's death, even if this is difficult, because these ceremonies provide closure to the older adult's life.

- Individuals may need professional assistance referral to accomplish grieving effectively.
- It is important to note that grief work is never completely finished, but the pain diminishes over time.

Widowhood

Several means exist to assist widows and widowers through the intensive grief period immediately after the loss of a spouse, including

- Support from family and health care professionals
- Widowhood support groups
- Clergy visitation
- Social services

- If the family had hospice services in place prior to the death of the spouse, support services continue for 1 year after the death.
- After the loss of a spouse, it is especially important for health care professionals to monitor the health status of the recently widowed older adult.
- It is during this period of intense grief that the widowed spouse may ignore self-care activities, become malnourished, not take medications appropriately, refuse social interactions, or indulge in substance abuse.
- The loss of intimacy after many years with a partner can seriously impact one's life and health.
- Physical and psychological closeness to someone is an important part of self-concept and self-esteem; widowhood after a long marriage can greatly impact one's self-image.
- The loss of a spouse and entrance into widowhood is generally perceived as a serious life event. It is classified as severe social stress that affects the health of the widowed individual.
- Older widowers tend to have more problems with household management after the loss of their wives, and older widows tend to experience increased financial burdens after the death of their husbands.

References

Hospice Association of America. (2007). Hospice facts and figures. Retrieved March 21, 2007, from http://www.nahc.org/HAA/2007HospiceFactsStatistics.pdf

Koenig, H. G. (2007). Religion and remission of depression in medical inpatients with heart failure/pulmonary disease. *Journal of Nervous and Mental Disease, 195*(5), 389–395.

Koenig, H. G., McCullogh, M., & Larson, D. B. (2001). *Handbook of religion and health*. New York: Oxford University Press.

Kubler-Ross, E. (1964). *On death and dying*. New York: Macmillan.

Matzo, M. L., & Sherman, D. W. (Eds.). (2006). *Palliative care nursing: Quality of care to the end of life*. New York: Springer Publishing.

Rowe, J. W., & Kahn, R. L (1997). Successful aging. *Aging, 10*, 142–144.

World Health Organization. (2005). *Definition of palliative care*. Retrieved June 6, 2005, from http://www.who.org

8

Acute and Chronic Physical Illnesses

As the older adult population continues to grow and life spans continue to increase, the number of chronic illnesses among older adults will also increase. These chronic conditions require effective disease management. It is estimated that, by the year 2030, approximately 150 million individuals will have a chronic condition, compared to 99 million in 1995 (Robert Wood Johnson Foundation, 1996). The Alliance for Aging Research (2002) reports that the average older adult has the following chronic medical conditions.

Cardiac and Peripheral Vascular Problems

Hypertension

Hypertension results from many nonmodifiable and modifiable risk factors and lifestyle behaviors. It is a serious risk factor for the development of many types of cardiovascular and renal diseases. (See Table 4.1 for a list of the JNC-VII criteria for blood pressure.) Hypertension is considered a silent killer because it has no signs and symptoms.

- Approximately one-third of people with hypertension are unaware that they have it.
- The American Heart Association (2005) estimates that, of those with hypertension, at least half are not on medication and about 25% more are on inadequate hypertensive therapy.
- The combination of diabetes and smoking together is more dangerous than either risk factor alone, and increases the risk of adverse events resulting from hypertension.

Nursing interventions for the treatment of hypertension include

- Diet and lifestyle modification

    - Exercise
    - Stress management

- Medication management

    - First-line therapy consists of thiazide diuretics such as hydrochlorothiazide (HCTZ®) or Diuril® and beta blockers such as atenolol (Tenormin®), labetolol (Normodyne®), or propranolol (Inderal®). Angiotensin-converting enzymes (ACE inhibitors) such as benazepril (Lotensin®) or captopril (Capoten®) calcium channel blockers such as amlodipine (Norvasc®) and diltiazem (Cardizem®) are used for first-line therapy only when diuretics and beta blockers are contraindicated.
    - Side effects of antihypertensive medications may include dry, persistent cough and erectile dysfunction.

Congestive Heart Failure

Congestive heart failure (CHF) is a chronic medical condition that results in acute medical crises; it occurs more commonly as people age.

- In the United States, approximately 4.8 million people have CHF, and each year, 400,000 new cases are diagnosed.
- Approximately one-half of older adults with CHF will die within 5 years of being diagnosed with the disease.
- The presentation and outcome of CHF are often influenced by the presence of comorbidity.

    - About 80% of all clients with CHF are age 65 and older.
    - CHF affects approximately 1 million older adults annually.
    - CHF is a multifaceted disease exacerbated by normal changes in the heart that accompany aging.
    - CHF commonly occurs when the pumping ability of the heart is impaired and it can no longer deliver adequate blood circulation to supply the body's metabolic requirements.
    - CHF may be used to refer to either left ventricular failure or right ventricular failure. The pathology in most older adults is left ventricular dysfunction.

- CHF is often caused by a myocardial infarction and coronary artery disease.
- Other causes of CHF include
  - Valvular dysfunction
  - Arrhythmias
  - Infections
  - Rheumatic heart disease
  - Hyperthyroidism
  - Anemia
  - Excess salt and fluid intake
  - Steroid administration
  - The discontinuation of cardiac medications
- The typical presentation of CHF in older adults includes the sudden development of
  - Shortness of breath
  - Dyspnea with exertion
  - Fatigue
  - Weakness
  - Alteration in function
  - Change in cognition
  - Pedal edema
  - Fluid in lungs
- Other symptoms may include
  - Diaphoresis
  - Tachycardia
  - Palpitations
  - Anorexia
  - Insomnia
- Normal and pathological aging changes may make the early assessment and treatment of CHF difficult.
  - Pedal edema or weight gain due to CHF may be confused with normal pedal edema that occurs with aging or the side effects of steroid treatment for chronic obstructive pulmonary disease.
  - Altered cough reflex may prevent early detection of pulmonary changes.
  - Chest pain or tightness, fatigue, general weakness, a nonproductive cough, and insomnia may be commonly attributable to other conditions of aging and orthopnea.

Nurses play an important role in identifying early symptoms of CHF through awareness of common signs and symptoms in older adults. Effective management of CHF in older adults includes

- Education about
  - Self-care—alternating periods of activity with rest
  - Low-salt or sodium-restricted diets

- Medication administration involving a combination of angiotensin-converting enzyme (ACE) inhibitors, digoxin, and diuretics and ACE inhibitors such as benazepril (Lotensin®) or captopril (Capoten®)

- Early identification of symptoms

  - Administration of diuretics to decrease cardiac workload. Without further symptoms, and adequate urinary output, older adults may be evaluated for several hours in the emergency department, home, or outpatient facility and then discharged.
  - The persistence of symptoms or failure to reduce cardiac output requires further treatment and hospitalization.

Angina and Myocardial Infarction

Angina occurs in approximately 13.7% of women and 21% of men aged 65 to 69.

- The *Merck Manual of Geriatrics* (Beers & Berkow, 2000) reports that myocardial infarction (MI) occurs in approximately 35% of older adults, and 60% of hospitalizations due to acute MI occur in persons 65 years and older. Moreover, 38% of women and 25% of men will die within 1 year of their MI (American Heart Association, 2008).
- A variety of factors can precipitate angina and MI among older adults, the most common of which is coronary artery disease.
- Other causes of MI include

  - Alular dysfunction
  - Arrhythmias
  - Infections
  - Rheumatic heart disease
  - Hyperthyroidism
  - Anemia
  - Excess salt and fluid intake
  - Steroid administration
  - Discontinuation of cardiac medications

- Angina results from a lack of oxygen supply to the heart muscle due to reduced blood flow around the heart's blood vessels.
- Angina is the most common symptom of myocardial ischemia and is experienced commonly among older adults with coronary artery disease.
- Myocardial infarction is a serious, sudden heart condition usually characterized by varying degrees of chest pain or discomfort, weakness, sweating, nausea, and vomiting, sometimes causing loss of consciousness.
- MI occurs when a part of the heart muscle dies because of sudden total interruption of blood flow to that area.
- The classic clinical presentation of MI regardless of gender results in pain.

- The pain and dysrhythmias of MI are often more serious in older adults than in younger clients as a result of both normal and pathological aging changes.
- Older adults may not exhibit normal signs of MI, such as

    - Crushing, radiating chest pain
    - Gray or cyanotic skin
    - Diaphoresis
    - Severe anxiety
    - Nausea and vomiting
    - Hiccoughs

- In older adults, symptoms of MI may be insidious or vague (silent heart attack), because older adults may:

    - Be reluctant to complain
    - Lack communication ability to complain
    - Have post-stroke aphasia
    - Have dementia

- Some older adults may attribute the symptoms of angina and MI to

    - Normal aging changes
    - Symptoms of other disease processes

- Older adults may not have chest pain but may complain about any combination of

    - Pain in the back, shoulder, jaw, or abdomen
    - Diminished level of consciousness or acute confusion
    - Nausea and vomiting
    - Hypotension
    - Dizziness or syncope
    - Transient ischemic attack
    - Cerebral vascular accident
    - Weakness
    - Fatigue
    - Falls
    - Restlessness
    - Incontinence

Nurses play an important role in identifying early symptoms of angina and MI. Because both of these diseases may present as pain among older adults, attention to pain complaints must be considered seriously and proper assessment implemented.

- Nurses' beliefs that pain is a natural and expected part of aging is among one of the most prevalent myths that prevent appropriate treatment of angina and MI among older adults.
- Many older adults tend to hesitate to report pain because they think nothing can be done to manage the pain and/or they are afraid to bother the nurse.

- Objective pain is aided by the presence of many standardized tools for assessing pain in older adults. A frequently used measure of pain evaluation is a numeric rating scale in which clients are asked to indicate the pain they are experiencing on a scale of 1 to 10, with 1 being very little pain and 10 being the worst pain imaginable.
- After pain complaints are validated, further symptoms of angina and MI should be evaluated with the interdisciplinary team using

  - Electrocardiograms
  - Cardiac enzyme evaluation

- MIs are medical emergencies and must be managed accordingly.
- Drug therapy for chronic angina usually involves

  - Daily application of nitroglycerin patches (Nitrodisc®, Nitro-Dur®) to enhance perfusion to the cardiac vessels
  - Maintenance of sublingual nitroglycerin pills (Nitrostat®, Nitrolingual®) in the case of angina. Proper teaching regarding the application of patches and the administration of sublingual nitroglycerin is needed
  - Lipid-lowering medications known popularly as statins, which are often effective in reducing further occlusion of the cardiac vessels
  - Assessing cholesterol levels in clients within the normal range in order to reduce morbidity and mortality among this population
  - Selective beta-blocker medications such as acebutolol (Sectral®) and atenonol (Tenormin®), which also may be prescribed to prevent MI in patients with angina

- Nurses may also implement programs of

  - Weight loss for obese clients
  - Physical activity
  - Low-cholesterol and low-sodium diets

Peripheral Vascular Disease

Peripheral vascular disease (PVD) is a broad term that refers to altered circulation in the extremities—usually the legs—resulting from poor vascularization over many years.

- Risk factors for PVD include

  - Diabetes
  - Smoking
  - High-fat diets
  - Sedentary lifestyle

- Intermittent claudication refers to vascular-related pain that develops in the muscles of the legs while walking.

  - Symptoms may be misattributed to arthritis or neuropathy.
  - PVD is assessed by the amount of distance ambulated before the onset of pain.

- Surgical procedures may be available to improve circulation in the case of disabling PVD.
- Exercise has been found to be effective when tolerated to promote collateral circulation.
- Deep vein thrombosis occurs when a blood clot, or thrombus, develops in the large veins of the legs and is a major risk of immobility after surgery.
  - DVT is characterized by acute onset of pain and edema in the affected extremity.
  - Because a clot may become free and clog a major artery, such as a pulmonary artery, DVTs are medical emergencies and should be treated accordingly with surgery and/or clot-dissolving medications.
  - Patients at high risk may continue to remain on Coumadin and should be counseled to wear antiembolitic stockings.

Respiratory Problems

Pneumonia

Pneumonia is the leading cause of death from infectious disease in the United States and the overall sixth leading cause of death in the United States (Institute for Clinical Systems Improvement, 2003). The death rate from pneumonia is especially high among older adults who have had surgery or mechanical ventilation.

- Normal changes of aging such as lowered immune status impact pneumonia as do changes in respiratory function, including
  - Altered cough reflex
  - Diminished airway clearance
- Further risk factors for pneumonia are the presence of chronic diseases and conditions such as
  - Chronic obstructive pulmonary disease
  - Congestive heart failure
  - Gastroesophageal reflux disease
  - Impaired swallowing
  - Tube feeding
  - Impaired mobility
  - Alterations in levels of nutrition
- The traditional symptoms of pneumonia are often absent or difficult to assess among older adults. These symptoms include
  - Cough
  - Fever
  - Dyspnea
  - Purulent sputum
  - Pleuritic chest pain

- Most older adults with pneumonia have a presentation of disease that consists of

  - Anorexia
  - Confusion, delirium, or change in behavior
  - Altered functional abilities
  - Decompensation of underlying illnesses

- Nursing interventions for the treatment of pneumonia include

  - The administration of medications aimed at destroying the causative organism or virus
  - Proper diet
  - Hydration
  - Treatment of fever and discomfort with acetaminophen or NSAIDs
  - Respiratory therapy such as postural drainage
  - Evaluation of complications that require follow-up or further therapy, including

    - Dyspnea
    - Worsening cough
    - Onset or worsening of chills
    - Fever occurring more than 48 hours after drug therapy is started
    - Intolerance of the medications

Influenza

- Influenza, commonly known as the flu, is a contagious viral disease that frequently infects the population in the winter months.
- The Centers for Disease Control (2007a) reports that between 10% and 20% of the U.S. population is infected with the flu each year.
- The flu is often only a mild disease in healthy children and adults, manifesting symptoms such as fever, sore throat, dry cough, headache, and aching muscles.
- Older adults are more likely to develop life-threatening complications from the flu, such as

  - Changes in mental status
  - Dehydration
  - Pneumonia
  - Extreme tiredness

- Each year, approximately 36,000 U.S. residents die from influenza, and 114,000 are hospitalized from the disease (Centers for Disease Control, 2007a).
- Older adults may present with flu symptoms differently from their younger counterparts.
- In older adults, the classic symptoms of cough, congestion, nausea, and vomiting may be absent or attributed to other disease processes.
- Older adults with the flu may present with acute confusion or delirium.

- Nursing interventions include

  - Nutrition
  - Hydration
  - Rest

- Symptomatic treatment of the disease includes the use of fever reducers such as acetaminophen or ibuprofen and cough suppressants.
- Vaccination remains the most commonly used method of preventing and reducing the impact of the flu.
- Vaccination is required each year because the flu viruses change constantly and unpredictably.
- Medicare currently reimburses providers for annual influenza vaccinations.

Tuberculosis

Some characteristics of tuberculosis:

- Infectious disease caused by mycobacterium tuberulosis
- Spread through droplets
- Infection may be prevented by respiratory clearance mechanisms (50% from high carriers)
- Lodges in lung and results in tubercle
- Long latency period

The epidemiology of tuberculosis:

- One-third of the world's population is infected with latent disease (4% to 6% of U.S. residents).
- 8 to 10 million worldwide will develop active infections annually.
- It is primarily a disease of young adults, but the risk of tuberculosis among older adults is significantly increased in the institutionalized population.

Symptoms of tuberculosis:

- Fatigue
- Anorexia
- Weight loss
- Cough
- Night sweats
- Fever
- Chest pain
- May be peripheral involvement

Diagnosis of tuberculosis:

- PPD or Mantoux > 5mm or greater
- QuantiFERRON-TB (better at detecting latent infection and immunization with bacillus Calmette-Guérin)

- Chest X-ray
- Lab—acid fast bacilli (may take 3 to 8 weeks)
- Active and passive disease treatment
- Strong clinical suspicion
- Multiple drug treatment regimen with isoniazid, rifampin, pyrazinamide, and ethambutol

Obstructive Airway Disease

Obstructive airway diseases collectively rank as the fourth leading cause of death in the United States. Chronic bronchitis, asthma, and emphysema are the three major obstructive airway diseases that collectively represent chronic obstructive pulmonary disease (COPD) found prevalently among older adults.

- Chronic bronchitis is caused by the inflammation of respiratory passages and results in edema and the development of sputum that tends to make breathing very difficult and in some cases impossible.
- Asthma is manifested by the onset of bronchospasm, mucosal edema, and large amounts of sputum production.
- Asthma is on the rise in the United States; the incidence and death rates of the disease are increasing among all age groups, including older adults.
- Some older adults grow old with the disease and some experience new onset asthma in their later years.
- Emphysema results from damage to the alveoli (the functional units in the lungs), which results in a reduction in the lung tissue available for aeration (alveolar-capillary diffusion interface).
- Chronic obstructive pulmonary disease can be the result of many factors, including
  - Air pollution
  - Smoking
- Nursing interventions for chronic obstructive pulmonary disease vary, but the goals of all disease therapies are to
  - Maintain patent airways with the use of suction and medication.
  - Teach patients about the use of inhalers.
  - Teach patients about energy conservation.
  - Teaching safe and effective oxygen administration.
  - Administer steroid medications as needed to decrease airway inflammation.
  - Administer opioids that have been supported as safe and effective in reducing terminal dyspnea and respiratory distress at the end of life.

Gastrointestinal Problems

Gastroesophageal Reflux Disease

- Gastroesophageal reflux disease (GERD) occurs frequently in older adults as a result of improper closure of the lower esophageal sphincter.

- This leads to regurgitation of stomach acid into the esophagus, leading to erosion or metaplasia.
- GERD places older adults at higher risk for esophageal cancers.
- Risk factors of GERD include (Miller, 2007)

  - Diets high in fat, caffeine, chocolate, peppermint, and garlic
  - Alcoholism
  - Consumption of large meals
  - History of hiatal hernia
  - Smoking
  - Use of the following medications:

    - Calcium channel blockers
    - Nitrates
    - Nonsteroidal anti-inflammatories (NSAIDs)
    - Anticholinergics

- Signs and symptoms of GERD include

  - Foul taste in mouth
  - Heartburn
  - Nausea
  - Belching
  - Dry cough

- Treatment usually involves

  - Administration of proton pump inhibitors Nexium™, Pepcid™, or Protonix™
  - Diet modifications to avoid causative foods
  - Elevating the head of the bed
  - Smoking cessation

Hematological Problems

Anemia

Anemia is a pathological illness among older adults generally resulting from abnormal hemoglobin and hematocrit levels. Older adults with anemia must be assessed to determine the responsible pathology.

- Medications may cause anemia among older adults.

  - Proton pump inhibitors taken for more than 5 years decrease the amount of intrinsic factor available for B_{12} absorption, resulting in macrocytic anemia.

- Other risk factors for anemia include

  - Crohn's disease
  - Ulcers
  - Gastritis
  - Surgical procedures such as ileostomies or colectomies or small bowel resection

- Cancer
- Renal disease
- HIV
- Other diseases that decrease bone marrow production

- Assessment for anemia includes frequent evaluation of hemoglobin, hematocrit, and associated blood values specific to type of anemia.
- Treatment includes

  - Diets high in protein and iron
  - Vitamin supplementation

Genitourinary Problems

Urinary Tract Infections

Urinary tract infections are the most common type of infection among older adults and are caused by an accumulation of pathological bacteria in the urine. The rate of urinary tract infections increases significantly among the institutionalized elderly.

- The symptoms of urinary tract infections are

  - Incontinence
  - Increased confusion
  - Falls
  - Urinary frequency
  - Dysuria
  - Suprapubic discomfort
  - Fever
  - Costovertebral tenderness

- Diagnosis generally involves the collection of a urine specimen for culture and sensitivity.
- Antibiotic treatment should occur only in the presence of symptoms.

  - A short course of antibiotics is usually recommended. Prolonged treatment may result in vaginitis in older women.
  - Treatment for longer periods of time may be needed among the older population due to their decreased natural immune responses.

- In-dwelling catheters should be avoided when possible due to the increased risk of developing infections.

Sexually Transmitted Diseases

While health care providers are becoming increasingly knowledgeable regarding the unique needs of older adults, the sexuality of this population remains largely unrecognized. Nurses often ignore the sexuality of older adults during assessments, assuming that this aspect of human functioning is no longer applicable. The possibility of an older adult contracting a sexually transmitted disease (STD) is real; these diseases include

- Neisseria gonorrhorae (gonorrhea)
  - May be asymptomatic in women but painful in men
  - Screen with smear
  - Treatment:
    - Ceftriaxone
    - Ciprofloxacin
    - Levofloxacin
- Treponema palladium (syphilis)
  - May be asymptomatic in both men and women but they both may be carriers
  - Can result in late cardiovascular and neurological effects
  - Screening is complicated
  - Should test exposed individuals
  - Treatment includes antibiotics
    - Penicillin
- Chlamydia trachomates (chlamydia)
  - Over 15 strands of this virus
  - The most common sexually transmitted disease
  - Major risk factor for pelvic inflammatory disorder
  - May be asymptomatic in women but painful in men
  - Assessment includes a screen with smear (clean cervical os)
  - Treatment:
    - Azithromycin or doxcycline or ceftriaxone
- Herpes types 1 and 2
  - Genital herpes
  - One in five individuals has herpes
  - Spread through direct contact with lesions during sexual encounters
  - Screen for morphology of lesions
  - Treatment:
    - Acyclovir
    - Famciclovir
    - Valacyclovir (first episode, recurrence, and suppression regimens)
- Human papilloma virus
  - Group of more than 70 viruses that affect genital mucous membranes
  - May be asymptomatic
  - May be associated with some cancers
- Nurses must conduct sexual assessments on older adults with the same frequency as other system assessments.

8.1 PLISSIT Model of Sex Therapy

P	Obtain Permission from the client to initiate sexual discussion.
LI	Provide the Limited Information needed to function sexually.
SS	Give Specific Suggestions for the individual to proceed with sexual relations.
IT	Provide Intensive Therapy surrounding the issues of sexuality for that client.

Note. From Annon, J. (1976). The PLISSIT model: A proposed conceptual scheme for the behavioral treatment for sexual problems. *Journal of Sex Education Therapy. 2*(2), pp. 1–15.

- Lack of experience and general discomfort with sexuality among health care providers are often barriers to assessing and managing the sexuality needs of older adults.
- A model to guide sexual assessment and intervention of older adults is available (Exhibit 8.1) and has been widely used among younger populations.
- The assessment of older adults' sexuality should take place in a quiet area that affords clients necessary privacy.
- The establishment of a trusting relationship between the health care provider and client is essential.
- Nurses must be cautious to be respectful of older adults' sexual beliefs and practices and must prevent judgmental thoughts and comments.
- Appropriate history questions regarding sexuality include

  - Number and history of partners
  - Sexual practices
  - Physical signs and symptoms of sexual problems
  - Presence of problems
  - Level of satisfaction with current sexuality
  - Use of protection and precautions. In the older adult population, STDs such as syphilis, genital herpes, and hepatitis may remain from earlier years and be passed unknowingly to partners.

Cancer

- Although the presence of cancer is seen in all populations, the incidence and prevalence of cancer is disproportionate in the elderly population.
- Approximately 75% of all malignancies in the United States occur among older adults, who, at present, constitute about 13% of the population.
- Individuals aged 65 and older accounted for 56% of all cases of breast cancer and 80% of all prostate cancer in 2002.

- Advanced age is a risk factor for the development of cancer.
- Older adults are more likely to be diagnosed with cancer at an advanced stage when the cancer is less amenable to treatment and increased morbidity and mortality are more likely.
- Cancer diagnosis and mortality are strongly associated with race and socioeconomic status.
- For both older men and women, lung cancer is the leading cause of mortality.
- Lung cancer mortality rates are followed by prostate cancer and colorectal cancer for older men and breast cancer and colorectal cancer for older women.
- Ageism and myths of aging prevented older adults from being involved in clinical trials for new cancer treatments; health care providers often perceived this population to be at high risk for adverse effects from the negative effects of cancer therapy.
- More recently, older adults have begun to receive aggressive treatments for cancer and are tolerating these treatments well. While special consideration for the normal and pathological changes of aging must be made, older adults should be offered the same treatments available to younger populations.
- Nurses play an instrumental role in the primary and secondary prevention of cancer (see chapter 5, Health Promotion).
- Providing support and information during the diagnosis is essential in treatment decision making and promoting effective cancer outcomes and quality of life.

Prostate Cancer

- Of all men diagnosed with cancer each year, more than 30% will be diagnosed with prostate cancer.
- This rate is higher for African Americans (American Cancer Society, 2007).
- Prostate cancer is nearly 100 percent survivable if detected early (US Too! International, 2004).
- The availability of prostate-specific antigen testing for prostate cancer has greatly increased the detection and treatment of early-stage prostate tumors in older men.
- Treatment for prostate cancer includes the options of

  - Internal radiation (brachytherapy)
  - External beam radiation therapy
  - Radical prostatectomy
  - Active surveillance or watchful waiting
  - Hormonal therapy for late-stage disease

- Nurses will be involved in administering treatments aimed at reducing the symptomatology surrounding this disease as well as aiding treatment.

Breast Cancer

- Among older women, over 214,000 new cases of breast cancer were diagnosed in the United States in 2006, resulting in over 40,000 estimated deaths.
- Like prostate cancer in men, the risk of developing breast cancer increases with age among women.
- Breast self-examination and mammography are helpful in screening for breast cancer.
- The progression in lumpectomy and mastectomy procedures as well as new developments in radiation and chemotherapy treatments have sharply increased the survival rate for breast cancer for older women.
- The nursing role in screening and administering treatments for breast cancer is essential in promoting good outcomes for these older women clients.

Musculoskeletal Problems

Osteoarthritis and Degenerative Joint Disease

- Osteoarthritis (OA) is one of the most common chronic disorders among older adults.
- OA is the number one cause of pain among older adults.
- OA affects approximately 46.4 million Americans, 8.8% of whom report an arthritis-related disability (Centers for Disease Control, 2007b).
- OA can be a primary disorder or a secondary disorder resulting from a previous anatomic abnormality, injury, or procedure or from occupational factors.
- Nursing assessment for OA includes

  - The evaluation of pain, because this is the presenting symptom for most patients
  - Radiographic examination of the joints, which helps to aid in the diagnosis and staging of OA

- The nursing role for the treatment for OA is aimed at

  - Relieving pain and preserving or restoring function

- Pharmacological treatments frequently include

  - Nonsteroidal anti-inflammatory drugs (NSAIDs)
  - Acetaminophen
  - Narcotic pain relievers, when necessary

- Various complementary and alternative therapies aimed at reducing pain and improving function are used frequently among older adults with OA.

  - Vitamins C, D, and E have shown some evidence of reducing symptoms.
  - Ginger and glucosamine also have been used extensively by older adults to reduce arthritis-related pain.

- Nurses must exercise caution in the administration of nutraceuticals and provide teaching regarding the possible danger of these herbals because little is known about the interaction of these medications with prescription medications that are used to treat other diseases.
- Acupuncture is becoming a more popular nonpharmacological OA management strategy.

- Joint replacement among older adults with osteoarthritis is gaining in popularity.
- Hip replacement surgery is common and greatly decreases pain and improves mobility among older adults.

  - Prosthesis may become dislodged if early adduction of hip is sustained.

- These surgical procedures are used primarily to replace hip and knee joints that are dysfunctional because of the long-term effects of osteoarthritis.
- Older individuals in their 80s and 90s typically have these procedures.
- Although the rehabilitation may be long and intense, joint replacements bring new mobility and have the potential to greatly improve quality of life.

Osteoporosis

Osteoporosis is among the most common chronic diseases of older adulthood.

- Physiologically, osteoporosis results from a demineralization of the bone and is evidenced by a decrease in the mass and density of the skeleton.
- The most common areas of bone loss are the vertebrae, distal radius, and proximal femur.
- Osteoporosis affects approximately 44 million women and men aged 50 and older in the United States. It is estimated that this number will grow to over 52 million by the year 2010 (National Osteoporosis Foundation, 2003).
- In older adults with osteoporosis, the overall decline in bone mass weakens the bone, making it vulnerable to even slight trauma.
- Normal changes of aging in the sensory system and in neuromuscular coordination combine with medications and environmental factors to place older adults with osteoporosis at high risk for fall-related fractures.
- Fractures of the humerus and femoral neck are common, as are hip fractures in women over age 65.

  - Hip fractures result in greater morbidity and mortality among older adults than any other type of fracture.

- Fractures in older adults often place these individuals in a spiral of iatrogenesis, with an increased risk of impaired mobility, decubitus ulcers, pneumonia, and incontinence.

- Older individuals who are at highest risk for osteoporosis include

    - Small, thin women who have fair skin and light hair and eyes
    - Older adults with a family history of osteoporosis
    - Postmenopausal women
    - Women over age 65
    - Men over age 80

- Older individuals are at greater risk if they

    - Have diets low in calcium
    - Smoke
    - Consume excess alcohol
    - Drink caffeine
    - Lead sedentary lifestyles

- Older adults with osteoporosis may develop kyphosis late in the disease.

    - Kyphosis is a convex curvature of the spine that causes loss of height and chronic back pain as well as abdominal protuberance, gastrointestinal discomfort, and pulmonary insufficiency.

- Bone density screenings can detect bone loss for those at risk for developing osteoporosis. However, because there are often no symptoms of this disease, osteoporosis is seldom diagnosed until a traumatic fracture is sustained.
- Nursing interventions for the prevention of osteoarthritis include

    - Encouraging diets high in calcium (1,500 mg per day).
    - Advising a program of regular weight-bearing exercise.
    - Medications that have been shown to prevent further bone loss in those diagnosed with osteoporosis. Alendronate sodium (Fosamax®) taken once a week or risedronate (Actonel®) or raloxifene (Evista®) has been shown to prevent further bone loss and develop new bone mass.
    - Nursing interventions also might include fall-prevention strategies (see chapter 5).

Metabolic and Endocrine Problems

Diabetes Mellitus

- Diabetes mellitus (DM) is a chronic medical disease manifested by an increase in blood glucose levels.
- The Centers for Disease Control (2005) report that 17 million Americans have DM, and over 200,000 people die annually from diabetes-related complications.
- DM is often a silent killer; it is estimated that 5.9 million Americans are unaware that they have the disease. Due to better screening and educational efforts at the state and national levels, diagnosis rates for diabetes

increased 49% from 1990 to 2000, and they are expected to continue to rise (Mokdad et al., 2001).

- DM is a chronic metabolic disease characterized by a deficiency in the production and utilization of the pancreatic hormone insulin. In older adults, elevated blood glucose levels symptomatic of DM result from altered insulin availability.
- There are two different types of diabetes mellitus: type 1 and type 2.

  - Type 1 is also known as juvenile-onset DM or insulin-dependent DM.
  - Type 2 DM generally appears during adulthood and is known as adult-onset DM or, more commonly, non–insulin dependent diabetes mellitus (NIDDM).

- Diabetes mellitus is considered a risk factor for heart disease.

  - More than 80% of persons with DM die of heart or blood vessel disease.
  - Smoking drastically increases the risk of cardiovascular disease in diabetics by constricting already compromised blood vessels.

- Nursing interventions for diabetes must begin with a thorough assessment of blood glucose values and HgA1C levels, which provide short- and long-term insulin function indicators.
- The type of therapy should be tailored to the individual client's needs and issues.
- Self-management of NIDDM in the elderly includes

  - Diet
  - Medication

    - Oral hypoglycemics
    - Insulin therapy

  - Blood glucose monitoring
  - Foot examinations
  - Exercise

Immunologic Problems

Human Immunodeficiency Virus/Acquired Immune Deficiency Syndrome

- 10% to 20% of HIV infections occur in people aged 50 and older.
- This number is most likely low because of misdiagnosis and will continue to rise as the population of older adults grows.
- Older adults progress from HIV to AIDS more quickly than younger adults because of normal and pathological aging changes.
- Due to the normal and pathological changes of aging, symptoms of HIV and AIDS may go undetected.
- The awareness of the possibility of sexually transmitted diseases among older adults heightens the awareness of these potential disorders.

- When sexual history questions lead the nurse to believe that the older adult is sexually active, especially with more than one partner, diagnostic testing should be conducted.
- Symptoms of HIV among older adults mimic other disease symptoms and may include
  - Diarrhea
  - Enlarged lymph nodes
  - Fever
  - Flulike symptoms
  - Headache
  - Rash
  - Fatigue
  - Anorexia
  - Weight loss
- Because HIV is often transmitted simultaneously with other STDs, the ELISA test may be used to diagnose the presence of the HIV virus.
  - If this test is positive, the Western blot test may be conducted to confirm HIV infection.
  - Viral cultures may be used to confirm HIV infection.
  - CD4 and viral load testing to measure the number of T helper cells helps to stage the disease.
- Nursing interventions for older adults with HIV include
  - Maintenance of health and function
  - Medication administration and teaching
  - Antiretroviral agents and highly active antiretroviral agents (the use of three or more antiretroviral agents together)
  - Nucleoside/nucleotide reverse transcriptase inhibitors
  - Nonnucleoside reverse transcriptase inhibitors
  - Protease inhibitors
  - Fusion inhibitors
  - Teaching safe sex practices

Neurological Problems

Parkinson's Disease

Parkinson's disease (PD) is one of the most common neurodegenerative disorders affecting the elderly population. It occurs in 1 of every 100 persons over the age of 60.

- It is estimated that 3% of persons over the age of 65 have PD, suggesting that the occurrence of the disease increases with age.
- Parkinson's disease affects men more than women and Whites more than Blacks or Asian Americans.
- Age is the primary risk factor for PD and so the disease is of concern among older adults.

- PD is a neurodegenerative disorder of slow and insidious onset, where 70% to 80% of the dopamine-producing neurons in the brain are destroyed by the time symptoms are present.
- The causes of PD have not been determined.

   - The roles of environmental toxins, poisons, viruses, and medications have been implicated in the development of PD, and these causes continue to be investigated.
   - Some medications—including chlorpromazine and haloperiodol as well as reserpine, methyldopa, and metacolpramide—have been linked to the development of PD symptoms.

- There are no objective clinical markers for PD.
- The diagnosis of PD is typically determined by the presence of three motor signs:

   - Tremor
   - Rigidity
   - Bradykinesia

- In addition to these common signs and symptoms, clients with the disease may exhibit cues such as

   - Postural instability
   - Autonomic dysfunction
   - Drug-induced symptoms

- Symptom management is the primary focus of nursing care. Psychological, social, and spiritual support are needed as the disease progresses.

   - Treatment of PD generally combines levodopa with carbidopa (Sinemet®).
   - Because levodopa competes with protein absorption from the small intestine, effective timing of medication is essential.
   - As symptoms progress, a client's ability to perform activities of daily living decreases and the need for pharmacotherapy increases.
   - To avoid potential side effects, patients may choose nonpharmacological treatment options, delay medical treatment, and postpone potential discomfort from the unwanted side effects.
   - Physical and occupational therapy may help those with a shuffling gait. Focusing on the client's balance abilities and providing assistive devices where applicable is recommended.
   - Nutritional therapy is also essential when caring for patients with Parkinson's disease.
   - Immobility is a major contributor to constipation, and, therefore, it is important to assess the dietary needs of PD clients to prevent severe constipation.
   - Exercise is also extremely therapeutic for clients with PD. It decreases the risk of falls related to the disease and improves

      - Mobility
      - Flexibility

- Posture balance
- Overall function

Cerebral Vascular Accident

- Cerebral vascular accidents (CVAs), commonly known as strokes, are among the leading cause of chronic disability in the United States.
- The risk of CVA increases sharply with age; approximately 75% of new strokes and 88% of stroke deaths occur among those aged 65 and older.
- The symptoms of CVA include

  - Sudden-onset weakness or numbness in the face, leg, or arm on one side of the body
  - Changes in vision; the loss of vision in one eye
  - Difficulty speaking or understanding language
  - Sudden-onset severe headache and dizziness
  - Unexplained falls

- Risk factors for the development of CVA are similar to those of other cardiovascular diseases.

  - Smoking
  - Alcohol abuse
  - Obesity
  - Diabetes
  - Hypertension
  - Advanced age
  - African American racial background

- CVAs are caused by three distinct pathological processes that stem from risk factors for the disease.
- Effective auscultation of the carotid arteries for bruits (the sound of turbulent blood flow) during routine health assessments greatly enhances the early detection of occlusions in the vasculature and facilitates stroke prevention.
- A hemorrhage results when a blood vessel in the brain ruptures and part of the brain tissue dies.
- Emboli, or clots that form in one area of the body, may travel to the brain and cause brain death.
- The carotid arteries that carry oxygenated blood to the brain may become clogged and prevent blood flow, resulting in tissue death (ischemia).
- Older adults with and without risk factors for the CVA sometimes experience "little strokes" or warning strokes called transient ischemic attacks (TIAs).

  - TIAs are manifested by lack of consciousness for a period of time lasting from 20 minutes to 24 hours.
  - Reports of TIAs should be accompanied by a full assessment and the identification of risk factors and symptomatology for CVA.

■ A plan of care to prevent strokes from occurring in patients with TIAs must be implemented immediately.

■ Prevention of CVAs generally involves the facilitation of adequate blood flow to the brain.

■ Carotid endarterectomy procedures are often implemented (cleaning plaque from the carotid artery) to enhance blood flow to the brain and reduce the chance of an embolus breaking off from the plaque and moving to the cerebral vasculature.

■ CVAs may be best prevented by implementing nursing interventions to reduce risk factors such as obesity and hypertension with

■ Diet and nutritional management
■ Exercise and weight reduction
■ Blood pressure management
■ Administration of daily aspirin

■ When symptoms of a stroke are present, diagnostic testing is conducted, including

■ Computed tomography scan
■ Carotid or cerebral angiography
■ Plasminogen activator, a clot-dissolving drug, may be administered immediately (within a few hours of symptom onset)
■ The plasminogen activator can dissolve clots that may have caused the stroke and quickly restore blood flow to the brain, but it is not effective in

■ Hemorrhagic stroke
■ Ischemic stroke

■ Nursing care for patients with CVA focuses on stabilization of the client and rehabilitation to the highest possible functional level

Decubitus

Decubitus Ulcers

A decubitus ulcer, commonly known as a pressure sore or bed sore, results from prolonged pressure to an area of the skin against a bed or chair or from rubbing or friction.

■ One million new pressure ulcers are estimated to develop each year.
■ Both intrinsic and extrinsic risk factors result in the development of decubitus ulcers, including

■ Immobility (primary risk factor for development of decubitus/pressure ulcers
■ Infection
■ Incontinence
■ Dementia

- Malnutrition
- Diabetes
- Circulatory disorders
- Vascular impairment
- Edema
- Impaired sensation
- Transferring
- High pressure surfaces
- Sheering
- Exposure to urine or feces
- Circulation

- Decubitus ulcers are classified according to the severity of the wound, usually in four stages or types (see Table 8.1)
- The most effective nursing intervention for pressure ulcers is prevention
- Assessment of risk factors (see Table 8.2) enables nurses to identify and implement preventative measures to avoid the development of these wounds
- Preventative measures include

    - The use of pressure-relieving devices such as

        - Mattresses
        - Pads
        - Footwear

    - Proper body alignment—Rule of 30 or head of bed elevated 30 degrees
    - Regular and consistent skin assessment by knowledgeable nursing professionals with a reliable instrument will help to detect decubitus at an early, treatable stage (insert 8–4)
    - Turning and repositioning schedules
    - Eliminating risk factors for malnutrition and appropriate meal planning
    - Dietary supplements may be necessary for providing needed nutrition among chronically ill older adults

- Pressure ulcer treatments include

    - Daily care with recommended products is implemented according to wound stage.

        - Stage one ulcers (nonblanchable erythema) are protected from further damage with good hygiene and pressure relief; transparent dressings may be used.
        - Stage two ulcers are characterized by partial thickness skin loss involving epidermis, dermis, or both and generally are treated with occlusive dressings and reevaluated at regular intervals.
        - Stage three ulcers are characterized by full thickness skin loss and deep craters with or without undermining; utilize normal saline or other product dressings.

8.1 Pressure Ulcer Staging System

Pressure ulcer definition

A pressure ulcer is a localized injury to the skin and/or underlying tissue usually over a bony prominence, as a result of pressure, or pressure in combination with shear and/or friction. A number of contributing or confounding factors are associated with pressure ulcers; the significance of these factors is yet to be elucidated.

Pressure ulcer stages

Suspected deep-tissue injury

Purple or maroon localized areas of discolored intact skin or a blood-filled blister due to damage of underlying soft tissue from pressure and/or shear. The area may begin as tissue that is painful, firm, mushy, boggy, warmer, or cooler as compared to adjacent tissue.

Further description

Deep-tissue injury may be difficult to detect in individuals with dark skin. Evolution may include a thin blister over a dark wound bed. The wound may further evolve and become covered by thin eschar. Evolution may be rapid, exposing additional layers of tissue even with optimal treatment.

Stage I

Intact skin with nonblanchable redness of a localized area usually over a bony prominence. Darkly pigmented skin may not have visible blanching, but its color may differ from the surrounding area.

Further description

The area may be painful, firm, soft, warmer, or cooler as compared to adjacent tissue. Stage I may be difficult to detect individuals with dark skin. May indicate at-risk persons (a heralding sign of risk).

Stage II

Partial thickness loss of dermis presenting as a shallow open ulcer with a red-pink wound bed, without slough. May also present as an intact or open/ruptured serum-filled blister.

Further description

Presents as a shiny or dry shallow ulcer without slough or bruising.[a] This stage should not be used to describe skin tears, tape burns, perineal dermatitis, maceration, or excoriation.

Stage III

Full thickness tissue loss. Subcutaneous fat may be visible, but bone, tendon, or muscle is not exposed. Slough may be present but does not obscure the depth of tissue loss. *May* include undermining and tunneling.

(*continued*)

8.1 Pressure Ulcer Staging System (*continued*)

Further description

The depth of a stage III pressure ulcer varies by anatomical location. The bridge of the nose, ear, occiput, and malleolus do not have subcutaneous tissue, and stage III ulcers can be shallow. In contrast, areas of significant adiposity can develop extremely deep stage III pressure ulcers. Bone/tendon is not visible or directly palpable.

Stage IV

Full thickness tissue loss with exposed bone, tendon, or muscle. Slough or eschar may be present on some parts of the wound bed. *Often* includes undermining and tunneling.

Further description

The depth of a stage IV pressure ulcer varies by anatomical location. The bridge of the nose, ear, occiput, and malleolus do not have subcutaneous tissue, and these ulcers can be shallow. Stage IV ulcers can extend into muscle and/or supporting structures (e.g., fascia, tendon, or joint capsule) making osteomyelitis possible. Exposed bone/tendon is visible or directly palpable.

Unstageable

Full thickness loss in which the base of the ulcer is covered by slough (yellow, tan, gray, green, or brown) and/or eschar (tan, brown, or black) in the wound bed.

Further description

Until enough slough and/or eschar is removed to expose the base of the wound, the true depth and, therefore, stage cannot be determined. Stable (dry, adherent, intact without erythema or fluctuance) eschar on the heels serves as the body's natural (biological) cover and should not be removed.

Note. From *Updated Pressure Ulcer Staging 2007,* by the National Pressure Ulcer Advisory Panel, retrieved from http://www.npuap.org/pr2.htm; Copyright 2007, National Pressure Ulcer Advisory Panel, used with permission.
[a] Bruising indicates suspected deep-tissue injury.

Sensory Problems

Common Eye Diseases

Cataracts
- Result from accumulation of particles in the lens of the eye
- Have great impact on vision
- Previously have been untreatable
- Laser procedures to clear the lens and return vision to normal can be completed in approximately 1 hour and have few side effects

8.2 Braden Scale for Predicting Pressure Sore Risk

Patient's Name _____ Evaluator's Name _____ Date of Assessment

Sensory Perception Ability to respond meaningfully to pressure-related discomfort	**1. Completely Limited** Unresponsive (does not moan, flinch, or grasp) to painful stimuli, due to diminished level of consciousness or sedation. OR Limited ability to feel pain over most of body.	**2. Very Limited** Responds only to painful stimuli. Cannot communicate discomfort except by moaning or restlessness. OR Has a sensory impairment that limits the ability to feel pain or discomfort over half of body.	**3. Slightly Limited** Responds to verbal commands but cannot always communicate discomfort or the need to be turned. OR Has some sensory impairment that limits ability to feel pain or discomfort in one or two extremities.	**4. No Impairment** Responds to verbal commands. Has no sensory deficit which would limit ability to feel or voice pain or discomfort.				
Moisture Degree to which skin is exposed to moisture	**1. Constantly Moist** Skin is kept moist almost constantly by perspiration, urine, etc. Dampness is detected every time patient is moved or turned.	**2. Very Moist** Skin is often, but not always, moist. Linen must be changed at least once a shift.	**3. Occasionally Moist** Skin is occasionally moist, requiring an extra linen change approximately once a day.	**4. Rarely Moist** Skin is usually dry, linen only requires changing at routine intervals.				
Activity Degree of physical activity	**1. Bedfast** Confined to bed.	**2. Chairfast** Ability to walk severely limited or nonexistent. Cannot bear own weight and/or must be assisted into chair or wheelchair.	**3. Walks Occasionally** Walks occasionally during day, but for very short distances, with or without assistance. Spends majority of each shift in bed or chair.	**4. Walks Frequently** Walks outside room at least twice a day and inside room at least once every two hours during waking hours.				
Mobility Ability to change and control body position	**1. Completely Immobile** Does not make even slight changes in body or extremity position without assistance.	**2. Very Limited** Makes occasional slight changes in body or extremity position but unable to make frequent or significant changes independently.	**3. Slightly Limited** Makes frequent though slight changes in body or extremity position independently.	**4. No Limitation** Makes major and frequent changes in position without assistance.				
Nutrition Usual food intake pattern	**1. Very Poor** Never eats a complete meal. Rarely eats more than one third of any food offered. Eats two servings or less of protein (meat or dairy products) per day. Takes fluids poorly. Does not take a liquid dietary supplement. OR Is NPO and/or maintained on clear liquids or IVs for more than 5 days.	**2. Probably Inadequate** Rarely eats a complete meal and generally eats only about half of any food offered. Protein intake includes only three servings of meat or dairy products per day. Occasionally will take a dietary supplement. OR Receives less than optimum amount of liquid diet or tube feeding.	**3. Adequate** Eats over half of most meals. Eats a total of four servings of protein (meat, dairy products) per day. Occasionally will refuse a meal, but will usually take a supplement when offered. OR Is on a tube feeding or TPN regimen which probably meets most nutritional needs.	**4. Excellent** Eats most of every meal. Never refuses a meal. Usually eats a total of four or more servings of meat and dairy products. Occasionally eats between meals. Does not require supplementation.				
Friction and Shear	**1. Problem** Requires moderate to maximum assistance in moving. Complete lifting without sliding against sheets is impossible. Frequently slides down in bed or chair, requiring frequent repositioning with maximum assistance. Spasticity, contractures, or agitation leads to almost constant friction.	**2. Potential Problem** Moves feebly or requires minimum assistance. During a move, skin probably slides to some extent against sheets, chair, restraints, or other devices. Maintains relatively good position in chair or bed most of the time but occasionally slides down.	**3. No Apparent Problem** Moves in bed and in chair independently and has sufficient muscle strength to lift up completely during move. Maintains good position in bed or chair.					

Score: 15–18 at risk; 13–14 moderate risk; 10–12 high risk; 9 very high risk

Total Score

Glaucoma

- Results from a pathological accumulation of pressure in the internal chamber of the eye
- Requires the consistent use of pressure-relieving eye drops
- Lower levels of lighting may be needed to promote patient comfort
- Regular ophthalmological appointments for pressure readings are essential
- Surgical interventions are available when necessary

Common Ear Disease: Presbycusis

- High-pitched hearing loss that occurs commonly with aging.
- Makes it difficult to hear higher-pitched voices, such as those of women and children.
- Treatment is usually associated with amplifying sound with hearing aids.

  - Older adults sometimes do not like hearing aids because they are embarrassed about needing them and because they amplify all noises in the environment, further aggravating the hearing deficit.
  - Assess for cerumen impaction as a further complicating factor in the hearing impaired.
  - Face older adults when speaking to facilitate lip reading.
  - Do not shout.
  - Assess for the appropriateness of using alternate forms of communication, such as writing instructions.

References

Alliance for Aging Research. (2002). Medical never-never land. Retrieved August 10, 2007, from http://www.agingresearch.org/content/article/detail1698

American Cancer Society. (2007). Overview: Prostate cancer, how many men get prostate cancer? Retrieved July 18, 2007, from http://www.cancer.org/docroot/CRI/content/CRI_2_2_1X_How_many_men_get_prostate_cancer_36.asp?sitearea=

American Heart Association. (2005). Heart disease and stroke statistics. 2005 update. Retrieved April 23, 2008, from http://www.americanheart.org/downloadedheart/

American Heart Association. (2008). Facts about women and cardiovascular diseases. Retrieved March 21, 2008, from http://www.americanheart.org/presenter.jhtml?identifier=2876

Annon, J. (1976). The PLISSIT model: A proposed conceptual scheme for the behavioral treatment for sexual problems. *Journal of Sex Education Therapy, 2*(2), 1–15.

Beers, M. H., & Berkow, R. (Eds.). (2000). *Merck manual of geriatrics* (3rd ed.). Whitehouse Station, NJ: Merck Research Laboratories.

Braden Scale. Retrieved June 27, 2007, from http://www.bradenscale.com

Centers for Disease Control. (2005). Highlights in minority health, November 2003: National diabetes awareness month. Retrieved May 20, 2008, from http://www.cdc.gov/omhd/Highlights/2002&3/HNov03.htm

Centers for Disease Control. (2007a). Key facts about the flu. Retrieved July 18, 2007, from http://www.cdc.gov/flu/keyfacts.htm

Centers for Disease Control. (2007b). Arthritis data and statistics. Retrieved July 18, 2007, from http://www.cdc.gov/arthritis/data_statistics/index.htm

Institute for Clinical Systems Improvement. (2003). *Health care guideline: Community acquired pneumonia in adults.* Retrieved May 5, 2005, from http://www.icsi.org

Miller, S. K. (2007). Getting a grip on GERD. *American Nurse Today, 2*(6), 12–14.

Mokdad, A. H., Bowman, B. A., Ford, E. S., Vinicor, F., Marks, J. S., Koplan, J. P., et al. (2001). The continuing epidemics of obesity and diabetes in the United States. *Journal of the American Medical Association, 286,* 1195–1200.

National Osteoporosis Foundation. (2003). America's bone health: The state of osteoporosis and low bone mass. Retrieved July 18, 2007, from http://www.nof.org/advocacy/prevalence/index.htm

National Pressure Ulcer Advisory Panel. (2007). *Updated pressure ulcer staging 2007.* Retrieved March 23, 2008, from http://www.npuap.org/pr2.htm

Robert Wood Johnson Foundation. (1996). Chronic care in America: A 21st century challenge. Princeton, NJ: Author.

Us Too! International. (2004). Informed brochure. Retrieved January 16, 2005, from http://www.ustoo.org

9

Cognitive and Psychological Disorders

Introduction

- In older adults, three pathological cognitive and psychological conditions occur frequently that lead to cognitive impairment.
- These conditions are commonly known by those who care for the elderly as the three Ds: delirium, depression, and dementia.
- It is important to understand the incidence, prevalence, causes, and treatment of these disorders in order to implement appropriate treatment (see Table 9.1).
- Delirium, depression, and dementia occur from completely different disease processes.
- Yet they all tend to result in similar symptoms of cognitive decline.
- It is important to recognize the existence of these conditions in older adults, screen for them appropriately, and refer older adults for further evaluation and treatment at the earliest possible point of care.
- Early detection by experienced nurses will reduce the negative effects of depression, delirium, and dementia.

9.1 Comparison of the Clinical Features of Delirium, Dementia, and Depression			
Clinical feature	Delirium	Dementia	Depression
Onset	Sudden/abrupt; depends on cause; often at twilight	Insidious/slow and often unrecognized; depends on cause	Coincides with major life changes; often abrupt but can be gradual
Course	Short; diurnal fluctuations in symptoms; worse at night, in darkness, and on awakening	Long; no diurnal effects; symptoms progressive yet relatively stable over time; may see deficits with increased stress	Diurnal effects, typically worse in the morning; situational fluctuations in symptoms, but less than with delirium
Progression	Abrupt	Slow but uneven	Variable; rapid or slow but generally even
Duration	Hours to less than 1 month; longer if unrecognized and untreated	Months to years	At least 6 weeks; can be several months to years
Consciousness	Disturbed	Clear	Clear
Alertness	Fluctuates from stuporous to hyper-vigilant	Generally normal	Normal
Attention	Inattentive; easily distractible and may have difficulty shifting attention from one focus to another	Generally normal	Minimal impairment but is distractible
Orientation	Generally impaired; disoriented to time and place; should not be disoriented to person	Generally normal	Selective disorientation
Memory	Recent and immediate impaired; unable to recall events of hospitalization and current illness; forgetful, unable to recall instructions	Recent and remote impaired	Selective or "patchy" impairment; "islands" of intact memory; evaluation often difficult due to low motivation

(continued)

9.1	Comparison of the Clinical Features of Delirium, Dementia, and Depression (*continued*)		
Thinking	Disorganized; rambling, irrelevant, and incoherent conversation; unclear or illogical flow of ideas	Difficulty with abstraction; thoughts impoverished; judgment impaired; words difficult to find	Intact but with themes of hopelessness, helplessness, or self-deprecation
Perception	Perceptual disturbances such as illusions and visual and auditory hallucinations; misperceptions of common people and objects	Misperceptions usually absent	Intact; delusions and hallucinations absent except in severe cases
Psychomotor behavior	Variable; hypoactive, hyperkinetic, and mixed	Normal; may have apraxia	Variable; psychomotor retardation or agitation
Associated features	Variable affective changes; symptoms of autonomic hypo-hyperarousal	Affect tends to be superficial, inappropriate, and labile; attempts to conceal deficits in intellect; personality changes, aphasia, agnosia may be present; lacks insight	Affect depressed; dysphoric mood, exaggerated and detailed complaints; preoccupied with personal thoughts; insight present; verbal elaboration; somatic complaints; poor hygiene; and neglect of self
Assessment	Distracted from task; fails to remember instructions; frequent errors without notice	Failings highlighted by family; frequent "near miss" answers; struggles with test; great effort to find an appropriate reply; frequent requests for feedback on performance	Failings highlighted by individual; frequent "don't know" answers; little effort; frequently gives up; indifferent toward test; does not care or attempt to find answer

Note. From Braes, T., Milisen, K., & Foreman, M. D. (2007). Assessing cognitive function. In E. Capezuti, D. Zwicker, M., Mezey, T. T. Fulmer, D. Gray-Miceli, & M. Kluger (Eds.), *Evidence-based geriatric nursing protocols for best practice* (3rd ed., pp. 43–44). New York: Springer Publishing.

- Therapeutic nursing interventions to improve the care of older adults and reduce the impact of the three Ds include reminiscence and life review. These two successful techniques are appropriate for older adults at all cognitive levels.

  - "Reminiscence is a multifaceted, multipurpose, naturally occurring mental phenomenon manifested across the life span in a variety of forms and contexts. Life review is one of those forms of reminiscence but it differs in that it is more intense and has more depth" (Haight & Haight, 2007).
  - These techniques promote security among older adults by reviewing comforting memories.
  - Haight, Michel, and Hendrix (2000) found a positive effect of reminiscence on reducing depression.
  - Puentes (2002) states that reminiscence is usually directed by a listener using questions or topics.
  - The typical reminiscence session takes the form of a semistructured 45-minute to 1-hour meeting focusing on the facilitation of positive memories, patient histories, and storytelling. The process rather than the product is key.

Depression and Suicide

- The frequent experience of loss among the elderly was once used to explain the large incidence of depression among older adults.
- The suicide rate among older adults is higher than in any other age group.
- Situational life events may play a role in the development of depression but are not usually the only cause. Such situational life events include

  - Retirement
  - Relocation
  - Loss of spouse, friends, and family
  - Financial constraints
  - Illness

- Recent research on depression indicates that there is more to the development of depression than the experience of loss.
- The role of neurotransmitters in the development of depression among older adults also contributes to the development of depression in this population.
- Because of the many physiological changes that accompany aging, older adults are more susceptible to the effects of altered neurotransmission than any other age group.
- Older adults have the highest rate of depression, and the rate is even higher among older adults with coexisting medical conditions.
- 12% of older persons hospitalized for problems such as hip fracture or heart disease are diagnosed with depression.
- Rates of depression for older people in nursing homes range from 15% to 25%.

- Genetic factors may be significant, because depression is often seen in members of the same family.
- Women have a higher incidence of depression than men.
- There is a strong correlation between alcohol or drug abuse and depression, not only in the client but in his or her family as well.
- Women have higher rates of depression than men, and unmarried individuals with low support networks are at high risk for depression.
- Assessment for depression in older adults should include

  - A complete history, including family history and suicide attempts
  - Completion of a depression scale such as the Geriatric Depression Scale (see Exhibit 9.1).

- In addition to the possibility of suicide, complications of depression include

  - Amplification of pain
  - Delayed recovery from surgery and illness
  - Cognitive impairment
  - Malnutrition

- Treatment options for depression include psychotherapy, medication, and electroshock therapy. The various treatment options may be combined or used individually.
- Psychotherapy led by mental health professionals includes

  - Individual talk therapy
  - Family therapy
  - Group therapy

- Medication options include

  - Selective serotonin reuptake inhibitors (SSRIs): fluoxetine (Prozac®), paroxetine (Paxil®), and sertraline (Zoloft®)

    - SSRIs are a relatively new class of medications that work by inhibiting the reuptake of serotonin, thus increasing its concentration in the space between nerve cells.
    - These antidepressant medications have an overall lower side effect profile than their predecessor antidepressants, but they are not perfect.
    - The most common side effects of SSRIs are:

      - Nausea
      - Diarrhea
      - Insomnia
      - Dry mouth
      - Tremors

    - SSRIs are usually given in the morning right after breakfast.
    - Recent reports on SSRIs have shown that clients with Parkinson's disease (and possibly other tremulous disorders) may experience exacerbations of their condition to the point of inducing parkinsonian crisis.

9.1 Geriatric Depression Scale: Short Form

A. Five (or more) of the following symptoms have been present during the same 2-week period and represent a change from previous functioning; at least one of the symptoms is either (1) depressed mood or (2) loss of interest or pleasure.
Note: Do not include symptoms that are clearly due to a general medical condition or mood-incongruent delusions or hallucinations.

1. Depressed mood most of the day, nearly every day, as indicated by either subjective report (e.g., feels sad or empty) or observation made by others (e.g., appears tearful). *Note:* In children and adolescents, can be irritable mood.
2. Markedly diminished interest or pleasure in all, or almost all, activities most of the day, nearly every day (as indicated by either subjective account or observation made by others).
3. Significant weight loss when not dieting or weight gain (e.g., a change of more than 5% of body weight in a month) or decrease or increase in appetite nearly every day. *Note:* In children, consider failure to make expected weight gains.
4. Insomnia or hypersomnia nearly every day.
5. Psychomotor agitation or retardation nearly every day (observable by others, not merely subjective feelings of restlessness or being slowed down).
6. Fatigue or loss of energy nearly every day.
7. Feelings of worthlessness or excessive or inappropriate guilt (which may be delusional) nearly every day (not merely self-reproach or guilt about being sick).
8. Diminished ability to think or concentrate or indecisiveness nearly every day (either by subjective account or as observed by others).
9. Recurrent thoughts of death (not just fear of dying), recurrent suicidal ideation without a specific plan, or a suicide attempt or a specific plan for committing suicide.

B. The symptoms do not meet criteria for a Mixed Episode.
C. The symptoms cause clinically significant distress or impairment in social, occupational, or other important areas of functioning.
D. The symptoms are not due to the direct physiological effects of a substance (e.g., a drug of abuse or a medication) or a general medical condition (e.g., hypothyroidism).
E. The symptoms are not better accounted for by Bereavement (i.e., after the loss of a loved one); the symptoms persist for longer than 2 months; or are characterized by marked functional impairment, morbid preoccupation with worthlessness, suicidal ideation, psychotic symptoms, or psychomotor retardation.

Note. From Aging Clinical Research Center, Stanford University. Retrieved March 22, 2008, from http://www.stanford.edu/~yesavage/GDS.html

- Tricyclic antidepressants (TCAs): amitriptyline (Elavil®), imipramine (Tofranil®), and nortriptyline (Pamelor®)

  - TCAs are among the oldest forms of antidepressants.
  - They work by blocking the reuptake of various neurotransmitters, such as norepinephrine and serotonin.
  - This action allows the chemicals to remain in the synaptic junction (the space between the neurons) for a longer period of time.
  - The presence of these neurotransmitters aids in the feeling of well-being.
  - Tricyclic antidepressants are associated with the following side effects:

    - Dry mouth
    - Constipation
    - Tremors
    - Blurred vision
    - Postural hypotension
    - Sedation
    - Urinary retention
    - Because some of these side effects increase the client's risk for falls, they are usually administered just before bedtime
    - It is also essential that clients on these medications be placed on a fall-prevention program

- Monoamine oxidase inhibitors (MAOIs): phenelzine (Nardil®) and tranylcypromine (Parnate®)

  - Monoamine oxidase inhibitors are seldom used.
  - They work by blocking various subtypes of monamine oxidase, which is the chemical responsible for breaking down norepinephrine, serotonin, and dopamine.
  - Like the TCAs, these chemicals remain in the neuroleptic synapse.
  - Common side effects of MAOIs:

    - Orthostatic hypotension
    - Tachycardia
    - Edema
    - Dizziness
    - Agitation

  - It is imperative that clients taking MAOIs follow a strict diet low in tyramines (found in aged cheeses, for example) and avoid certain medications (such as those containing ergotamine).
  - Failure to follow these restrictions could precipitate a hypertensive crisis that is potentially life threatening (Bernstein, 1995).

- Atypical antidepressants do not fall into a specific drug category.

  - Trazadone (Desyrel®) inhibits serotonin reuptake.

- Bupropion (Buspar®) is a mild blocker of the reuptake of dopamine, norepinephrine, and serotonin.
- Side effects for both include

  - Dry mouth
  - Dizziness
  - Drowsiness
  - Nausea
  - Vomiting
  - Increased risk of seizures

- Electroconvulsive therapy (ECT)

  - ECT is used in clients who have treatment-resistant depression.
  - ECT is not the usual first-line treatment for depression at any age.
  - It is effective in clients age 65 and older and is sometimes safer than multiple medications taken over a long period of time.
  - Older adults may experience more memory loss for a period of time after the treatment.
  - ECT has changed dramatically over the years.
  - The client is given both an anesthetic and a muscle relaxant prior to this short treatment.
  - The client is awakened shortly after the procedure is completed.
  - There is usually some initial confusion and disorientation, but that eventually resolves.
  - ECT treatments are typically given every other day for 6 to 12 treatments. The results can be rapid and profound.

Relationship of Depression and Suicidal Ideation

- The depressed client has an increased risk of suicidal ideation.
- Approximately 15% of severely depressed people commit suicide.
- Depressed people have 30 times the suicide risk compared to the general population.
- Suicide among older adults is particularly common.
- People age 65 and older account for 12% of the population, but they commit almost 20% of all suicides.
- Women make more suicide attempts, but men complete their attempts three times more often.
- The most vulnerable group at risk for suicide are unemployed single men who live alone.
- Suicidal ideation is the phrase used to describe the thought process of thinking about suicide.
- Nurses should ask specifically whether the client is thinking of hurting or killing himself or herself.
- Research has shown that 80% of people who have committed suicide told someone about it first, often a primary care provider.
- If a person talks about suicide, he or she has active suicidal ideation, and action must be taken immediately.

- One should never leave a person with active suicidal ideation alone.
- If the person is not an inpatient, he or she should be taken to the nearest psychiatric center or emergency department.
- If an older adult refuses to go, the legal system has several options to help protect the suicidal person—call 911.
- If a suicide attempt appears imminent, the client is put on constant one-to-one monitoring.
- The client's primary health care professional should be notified immediately so that the need for drug therapy can be evaluated and initiated if indicated.
- All items that could be potentially used by the client to cause injury should be removed. These items include

  - Razors
  - Jewelry with pins or sharp points
  - Belts
  - Shoelaces
  - Eating utensils
  - Mirrors
  - Nails used to hang pictures on the walls
  - Nail files
  - Medications
  - Aerosol sprays
  - Paint

Dementia

- Decline in the cognitive function of older adults is a prevalent concern and a focus of study in the older population.
- While normal changes of aging result in a decrease in brain weight and a shift in the proportion of gray matter to white matter, the development of dementia is not a normal change of aging.
- Dementia is a general term used to describe over 60 pathological cognitive disorders that occur as a result of

  - Disease
  - Heredity
  - Lifestyle
  - Environmental influences

- Dementia has underlying organic causes, including

  - Vascular disease
  - Central nervous system infections
  - Cortical degeneration
  - Brain trauma
  - Metabolic or toxic disorders
  - Neurological disorders such as Alzheimer's disease or Parkinson's disease

- Memory losses are common to older adulthood, but they are often falsely labeled as dementia.
- Dementia is a chronic loss of cognitive function that progresses over a long period of time.
- Dementia, as defined by the Alzheimer's Association (1999), is a "loss of mental function in two or more areas such as language, memory, visual and spatial abilities, or judgment severe enough to interfere with daily life" (p. 8).
- A commonly used scenario to discriminate between normal memory loss and dementia is: If you lose your car keys, you simply experienced memory loss. If you find them and don't know what they are for, this may signal a cognitive problem.
- Essential features of dementia include short- and long-term memory loss associated with impairment in construct thinking, impaired judgment, and other disturbances of higher cortical function that may result in personality change, which may be manifested in

    - Difficulty coping with new situations
    - Excessive motor or verbal activity
        - Irritability
        - Restlessness
        - Resisting needed assistance
        - Hyperactivity
        - Wandering
        - Assaultiveness
        - Threatening gestures
        - Spitting
        - Physical destructiveness
        - Verbal abuse
        - Belligerence
        - Screaming
        - Swearing
        - Expressions of anger

- Alzheimer's disease (AD) is the most common type of dementia, making up over 50% of dementia cases.
    - The cause of AD is not known.
    - Two risk factors for the development of AD are
        - Advanced age
        - Family history of the disease

- Ten early warning signs of AD are
    - Misplacing items
    - Loss of initiative
    - Changes in personality
    - Poor judgment
    - Changes in mood or behavior
    - Disorientation to time and place
    - Memory loss that affects job skills
    - Difficulty performing familiar tasks

- Difficulty finding the right words
- Problems with abstract thinking

- Assessment of cognitive function to diagnose dementia:

  - A standardized cognitive assessment instrument such as the Mini-Cog (see Figure 4.1 in chapter 4) can be used.
  - Definitive diagnosis of all but multi-infarct dementia formerly was limited to postmortem brain autopsy.
  - Recent advances in computed tomography scans, magnetic resonance imaging, and, most importantly, positron emission tomography have improved the ability to diagnose Alzheimer's disease with more than 90% accuracy.
  - If older adults score low on screening instruments for cognitive impairments, they should be evaluated

    - for a comprehensive geriatric assessment to aide in the diagnosis of AD
    - to rule out delirium and depression as possible causes of altered cognitive functions

  - Working with older adults with cognitive disorders can be challenging and frustrating.
  - Assessments and care may need to be stopped to facilitate patient comfort and safety.
  - The focus is on maintaining function and independence as much as possible, while keeping the older adult safe.
  - Nurses who work with older adults are developing interventions to increase the quality of life for those who suffer from dementia.
  - These interventions include

    - Maintaining familiar environments to keep patients comfortable and safe
    - Necessary environmental manipulations such as camouflaging doors and installing door alarms
    - Applying wander guards
    - Providing safe wandering areas

- The Alzheimer's Association (2006) recommends the techniques shown in Table 9.2 for caring for older adults with dementia.
- Several medications known as cholinesterase inhibitors have been developed to increase the levels of acetylcholine in the brain and prevent further loss of cognitive function. These medications include

  - Donepezil (Aricept®)
  - Galantamine (Reminyl®)
  - Rivastigmine (Exelon®)
  - Tacrine (Cognex®)

- Memenda or memintine differs from the cholinesterase inhibitors but works well in combination with this classification of drugs and appears to be well tolerated.

9.2 Tips for Caring for Older Adults With Dementia		
Assess	**Intervene**	**Evaluate**
Identify the troublesome behaviors	*Explore potential solutions*	*Did your intervention help?*
▦ What was the behavior?	▦ Are there unmet needs of the person with dementia—is he or she sick, in pain, or sexually unfulfilled?	▦ Do you need to explore other potential causes and solutions to the behavior?
▦ What happened just before or after the behavior? Did something trigger it?	▦ Can you adapt the environment instead of the person?	
▦ What was your reaction?	▦ Can you change your reaction or approach to the behavior?	

Note. Adapted from Behaviors. (2006). Alzheimer's Association. Retrieved March 22, 2008, from http://www.alz.org/national/documents/brochure_behaviors.pdf

Delirium

▦ Delirium is defined as a transient state of global cognitive impairment (Foreman, 1993).

   ▦ Reduced ability to maintain attention to external stimuli and to shift appropriate attention to new external stimuli
   ▦ Disorganized thinking
   ▦ At least two of the following:

      ▦ Reduced level of consciousness
      ▦ Perceptual disturbances
      ▦ Disturbance of the sleep-wake cycle
      ▦ Increased or decreased psychomotor behavior
      ▦ Disorientation to person, place, or time
      ▦ Memory impairment

▦ These symptoms of delirium, commonly thought of as acute confusion, usually develop over a short period of time.
▦ Estimates of the incidence and prevalence of delirium in acute care settings show that approximately 16% of older adults experience this short-term cognitive disorder.
▦ Delirium is not a disease as much as a syndrome that may result from a variety of causes.
▦ The specific symptoms of delirium that separate it from dementia are

   ▦ Acute onset
   ▦ Fluctuating course

- Delirium may develop in both cognitively intact and cognitively impaired older adults.
- The cause of delirium is not fully known.
- Suggested risk factors for the onset of delirium:

  - Previous brain pathology
  - Decreased ability to manage change
  - Impaired sensory function
  - Presence of acute and chronic diseases
  - Changes in medications
  - Translocation
  - Cognitive impairment
  - Sensory impairment or deprivation
  - Comorbidity
  - Depression
  - Alcohol use
  - Physical restraints
  - Malnutrition
  - More than three medications
  - Urinary catheterization
  - Iatrogenic events

- Delirium has vast implications for older adults, their families, and the U.S. economy, including

  - Increased hospital stays
  - Failure to assess underlying and causative disease processes

- Prevention of delirium by risk factor minimization is essential.
- If delirium is assessed, treatment includes

  - Identification and removal of the cause
  - Keeping the older adult safe
  - Implementing fall and wandering interventions
  - Avoiding the use of restraints (physical and chemical) because this may exacerbate the delirium
  - Maintaining nutrition and hydration status
  - Providing a calm, soft-spoken approach to care
  - Frequently reassuring families of the temporary nature of this syndrome

References

Alzheimer's Association. (1999). Alzheimer's disease and related dementias fact sheet. Retrieved March 22, 2008, from http://www.alz.org/national/documents/brochure_basics ofalz_low.pdf

Alzheimer's Association. (2006). Behaviors. Retrieved March 22, 2008, from http://www.alz.org/national/documents/brochure_behaviors.pdf

Bernstein, J. A. (1995). Nonimmunologic adverse drug reactions: How to recognize and categorize some common reactions. *Postgraduate Medicine, 98,* 120–126.

Braes, T., Milisen, K., & Foreman, M. D. (2007). Assessing cognitive function. In E. Capezuti, D. Zwicker, M. Mezey, T. T. Fulmer, D. Gray-Miceli, & M. Kluger (Eds.), *Evidence-based geriatric nursing protocols for best practice* (3rd ed., pp. 41–56). New York: Springer Publishing.

Foreman, M. D. (1993). Acute confusion in the elderly. *Annual Review of Nursing Research, 11,* 3–30.

Haight, B. K., & Haight, B. S. (2007). *The handbook of structured life review.* Baltimore: Health Professions Press.

Haight, B. K, Michel, Y., & Hendrix, S. (2000). The extended effects of the life review in nursing home residents. *The International Journal of Aging and Human Development, 50,* 151–168.

Puentes, W. J. (2002). Simple reminiscence: A stress-adaptation model of the phenomenon. *Issues in Mental Health Nursing, 23*(5), 497–511.

10

Medication

Polypharmacy

- The use of prescription, nonprescription, over-the-counter (OTC), and herbal medications among older adults is widespread.
- The availability of multiple and effective medications to treat the numerous diseases among older adults undoubtedly plays an instrumental role in the increasing life span of this population.
- Excessive and inappropriate medication among older adults remains one of the most prevalent problems in the older population (Morley, 2003).
- In the United States, older adults spend approximately $3 billion annually on prescription medications.
- As older adults age, the number of prescription medications increases.
- The Alliance for Aging Research (2002) reports that the average older adult uses five prescription drugs and many over-the-counter medications.

Pharmacokinetics and Pharmacodynamics

- Pharmacokinetics is the study of drug absorption, distribution, protein binding, hepatic metabolism (biotransformation), and renal excretion.
- Pharmacodynamics is the study of drug effects at the receptor level.
- Normal changes of aging and pathological illness often influence pharmacokinetics and pharmacodynamics among older adults. These changes are summarized in Table 10.1.
- The four pharmacokinetic mechanisms—absorption, distribution, metabolism, and elimination—are also influenced by acute and chronic illnesses common in older adulthood, which may further slow or impair the ability of organ systems to absorb, distribute, metabolize, and excrete medications.

10.1 Pharmacokinetic Changes With Aging	
Pharmacokinetics	Changes in older adults
Drug absorption	▪ Increase in gastric pH and a change in the amount of fluid in the stomach ▪ Decrease in time required for emptying stomach contents ▪ Takes stomach longer to move nutrients across the membrane ▪ Increased time needed for medications to become effective ▪ Increased time may also increase amount of medication absorbed ▪ Vitamins A and C may be more readily absorbed
Drug distribution	▪ Reduced lean body mass ▪ Increase in percentage of body fat ▪ Total body intracellular and extracellular water decreases by 15% ▪ Alterations in plasma protein binding ▪ Cardiac output declines by 1% every year ▪ Blood flow to the liver declines from 0.3% to 1.5% a year
Drug metabolism	▪ Reduced blood flow to the liver ▪ Decrease in functional liver cells ▪ The enzymes used to break down medicines are reduced
Drug elimination	▪ Reduction in the mass and a reduction in the number and size of the nephrons ▪ Reduced glomerular filtration rate ▪ Decreased renal tubular secretion ▪ Increased medication half-life

- These changes affect how medications are

  - Absorbed through the gastrointestinal track, skin, or musculature.
  - While older adults experience many anatomical and physiological changes throughout life, there is currently little evidence to support the notion that normal aging significantly impacts drug absorption.
  - A substantial prevalence of nutritional deficiencies exists among older adults.
  - Diseases that may impact drug absorption include

    - Achlorhydria, a disease that reduces the acidity of the stomach, which may make it difficult to dissolve medications for absorption
    - Gastroesophageal reflux disease
    - Surgery to the stomach or small intestine

  - Distributed via the circulatory system

    - Total body intracellular and extra cellular water decreases by as much as 15% among older adults.

    - This reduces the distribution of water-soluble medications and increases the amount of fat soluble medications.
    - Lean body mass is reduced in older adults.
    - The proportion of fat tissue increases with age from 18% to 36% in men and from 36% to 48% in women between the ages of 20 and 80.

    - Fat-soluble medications such as barbiturates, phenothiazines, benzodiazepines, and phenytoin have the tendency to accumulate in the increased fat distribution of older adults, resulting in a prolonged half-life of these medications.
    - Alterations in plasma protein binding that may occur as part of the normal aging process could alter the distribution of a medication significantly, as well as change the half-life of a medication and disrupt the steady flow of medication needed for disease management.
    - Cardiac output, which declines by about 1% each year after the age of 30, has the potential to alter medication distribution.
    - Pathological illness affecting the circulatory system (i.e., diabetes) may impact medication distribution.

  - Metabolized by the bodily organ systems

    - Although medication metabolism depends on adequate liver function, that function is difficult to determine.
    - In the absence of diagnosed liver disease, it can be challenging to predict how medications will be metabolized among the elderly.
    - The following factors potentially affect liver function and reduce the metabolism of medications:

      - Multiple medications
      - Alcohol use

- Caffeine use
- Smoking
- Poor nutrition
- Multiple disease processes

- Eliminated from the body through the kidneys

  - Elimination of medications among older adults is one of the most well-studied and predictable age-related changes in medication pharmacokinetics.
  - Creatinine clearance is not be the most reliable measure of renal function and elimination of medications among older adults.
  - A more sensitive measure of medication elimination of older adults incorporates several variables such as body build or weight, age, and gender.

Adverse Drug Reactions and Side Effects

- Changes of aging and pharmacodynamics as well as the presence of disease and the numerous prescription and OTC drugs taken by older adults (polypharmacy) put this population at high risk for developing adverse reactions to drugs.
- Older adults are estimated to be at two to three times higher risk for adverse reactions to medications than their younger counterparts.
- Drug-drug interactions

  - Drug-drug interactions are defined as the combination of two or more drugs such that the potency or efficacy of one drug is significantly modified by the presence of another.
  - Despite the fact that the average older adult has three chronic diseases (Alliance for Aging Research, 2002), the number of older adults in clinical trials for new medications remains quite low.
  - Consequently, information on the appropriate dosing, side effects, and medication interactions is not available to guide the use of these medications among the elderly.

- Drug-disease interactions

  - Older adults with certain diseases may have drug intolerance, such as

    - Hypertension
    - Congestive heart failure
    - Diabetes
    - Renal failure

  - These drug-disease interactions may necessitate discontinuation of a medication or finding an alternative that does not impact other disease processes.

- Drug-nutrient interactions
  - Drugs have been shown to impact the nutritional status of older adults in the following ways:
    - Medications tend to impact appetite.
    - Medications may affect the absorption, distribution, metabolism, and elimination of nutrients.
    - Nutrients may impact the absorption, distribution, metabolism, and elimination of drugs.
  - Older adults are at higher risk for drug-nutrient interactions because of
    - Normal and pathological aging changes
    - Higher rates of alcoholism among the elderly
    - Use of restricted diets to treat disease
    - Use of nutritional supplements
  - Administering medications via tube feedings creates a risk of drug-nutrient interactions.
  - Certain nutrients are excreted more quickly if they interact with medications such as diuretics (thiazide, for example).
  - To reduce the risk of drug-nutrient interactions, medications should be administered with water.

Compliance Issues

- About half of all patients take their medications as prescribed upon leaving the physician's office. The other half take the medications incorrectly or not at all.
- Reasons for noncompliance with medication regimes include
  - Failure of health care professionals to give clear instructions on use of the medication
  - Inability to afford medication
  - Forgetfulness by the client
  - Inability to understand complex medication dosing
  - Conflict beliefs about healing
- Nursing interventions that may be helpful in enhancing medication adherence include
  - Assessment of understanding and beliefs regarding medications
  - Teaching regarding the recommended treatment regimen
  - The use of containers that are easily opened
  - Bold labeling of medications

References

Alliance for Aging Research. (2002). *Ageism: How healthcare fails the elderly.* Retrieved October 16, 2003, from http:/www.agingresearch.org

Morley, J. (2003). Editorial: Hot topics in geriatrics. *Journal of Gerontology Medical Sciences, 58A,* 30–36.

11

Special Issues

Pain

- Pain is a major problem for older adults and those who care for them.
- Pain has major implications for older adult health, functioning, and quality of life.
- Flaherty (2007) reports that 25% to 50% of community-dwelling older adults and 45% to 85% of nursing home residents have untreated pain.
- The number one cause of chronic pain among older adults is osteoarthritis.
- The American Geriatrics Society Panel on Chronic Pain in Older Persons (1998) states that there are many poor consequences of pain, including

  - Depression
  - Decreased socialization
  - Sleep disturbances
  - Impaired ambulation
  - Increased health care utilization and costs

- Despite the prevalence and impact of pain on older adults, many barriers prevent effective pain assessment and management:
  - Nurse's beliefs that pain is a natural and expected part of aging
  - Older adults' hesitancy to report pain
  - Normal and pathological changes of aging that affect the presentation of pain in older adults
  - The unavailability of objective biological markers of pain
- The most effective method on which nurses must rely to assess pain is the patient's self-report.
- Many standardized tools are available for assessing pain in older adults (see Figure 11.1).
  - A numeric rating scale on which the client is asked to choose a number from 1 to 10 that best describes the pain he or she is experiencing, with 1 being very little pain and 10 being the worst pain imaginable.
  - Visual Analogue Scales (VAS), which are straight horizontal 100-mm lines with verbal pain descriptors on the left and on the right sides.
  - The Faces Scale, which depicts facial expressions on a scale from zero to six, with zero = smile and six = crying grimace.
- Determining the right tool for each patient is necessary to utilize these objective measures effectively. These scales may be used for baseline and subsequent pain assessments to evaluate the effectiveness of treatment.

11.1 Faces pain scale. In the following instructions, say "hurt" or "pain," whichever seems right for a particular patient.

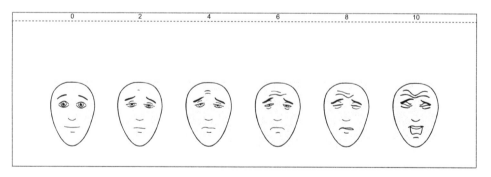

"These faces show how much something can hurt. This face [point to left-most face] shows no pain. The faces show more and more pain [point to each from left to right] up to this one [point to right-most face]—it shows very much pain. Point to the face that shows how much you hurt [right now]."

Score the chosen face 0, 2, 4, 6, 8, or 10, counting left to right, so 0 = no pain and 10 = very much pain. Do not use words like *happy* and *sad*. This scale is intended to measure how patients feel inside, not how their face looks.

Source: Pediatric Pain Sourcebook. (2007). Faces Pain Scale. Retrieved March 23, 2008, from http://painsourcebook.ca/pdfs/pps92.pdf

- For older adults with cognitive impairments, clients may not be able to verbalize pain appropriately and need special assessment (see Figure 11.2). In these patients, pain behaviors may include

  - Yelling out
  - Wandering
  - Repetitive behavior
  - Aggressive behavior

- Pain treatment includes

  - Treatment of the underlying cause of pain
  - Pharmacological pain management following a "start low and go slow" protocol (American Geriatrics Society, 1998)

    - Acetaminophen
    - Nonsteroidal anti-inflammatory drugs (NSAIDs)
    - Opioids

  - Collaborative pain medications, such as

    - Antidepressants
    - Anticonvulsants
    - Anxiolytics
    - Nonpharmacological pain management strategies
    - Exercise
    - Educational and cognitive therapy
    - Massage
    - Acupuncture
    - Therapeutic touch
    - Reiki
    - Reflexology

Sexuality

- One of the most prevalent myths of aging is that older adults are no longer interested in sex.
- A survey of 3,005 U.S. older adults found that sexual activity was reported in 73% of adults age 57 to 64, 53% of adults age 65 to 74, and 26% of adults age 75 to 84 (Lindau et al., 2007).
- The need to maintain one's sexuality and sexual function should be as highly valued as other physiological needs.
- Nurses and other health care providers do not regularly assess sexuality, and few intervene to promote the sexuality of the older population because of

  - Lack of knowledge
  - Lack of education regarding sexuality in aging
  - General inexperience and discomfort with the issue

- The fulfillment of sexual needs may be just as satisfying for older adults as it is for younger people.

11.2   Pain Assessment in Advanced Dementia (PAINAD) Scale.

Items[a]	0	1	2	Score
Breathing independent of vocalization	Normal	Occasional labored breathing. Short period of hyperventilation.	Noisy labored breathing. Long period of hyperventilation. Cheyne-Stokes respirations.	
Negative vocalization	None	Occasional moan or groan. Low level speech with a negative or disapproving quality.	Repeated troubled calling out. Loud moaning or groaning. Crying.	
Facial expression	Smiling or inexpressive	Sad. Frightened. Frown.	Facial grimacing.	
Body language	Relaxed	Tense. Distressed pacing. Fidgeting.	Rigid. Fists clenched. Knees pulled up. Pulling or pushing away. Striking out.	
Consolability	No need to console	Distracted or reassured by voice or touch.	Unable to console, distract or reassure.	
			Total[b]	

Breathing

1. Normal breathing is characterized by effortless, quiet, rhythmic (smooth) respirations.
2. Occasional labored breathing is characterized by episodic bursts of harsh, difficult, or wearing respirations.
3. Short period of hyperventilation is characterized by intervals of rapid, deep breaths lasting a short period of time.
4. Noisy, labored breathing is characterized by negative-sounding respirations on inspiration or expiration. They may be loud, gurgling, or wheezing. They appear strenuous or wearing.
5. Long period of hyperventilation is characterized by an excessive rate and depth of respirations lasting a considerable time.
6. Cheyne-Stokes respirations are characterized by rhythmic waxing and waning of breathing from very deep to shallow respirations with periods of apnea (cessation of breathing).

Negative Vocalization

1. None is characterized by speech or vocalization that has a neutral or pleasant quality.
2. Occasional moan or groan is characterized by mournful or murmuring sounds, wails, or laments. Groaning is characterized by louder-than-usual inarticulate involuntary sounds, often abruptly beginning and ending.
3. Low-level speech with a negative or disapproving quality is characterized by muttering, mumbling, whining, grumbling, or swearing in a low volume with a complaining, sarcastic, or caustic tone.
4. Repeated troubled calling out is characterized by phrases or words being used over and over in a tone that suggests anxiety, uneasiness, or distress.

5. Loud moaning or groaning is characterized by mournful or murmuring sounds, wails or laments much louder than usual. Loud groaning is characterized by louder-than-usual inarticulate involuntary sounds, often abruptly beginning and ending.
6. Crying is characterized by an utterance of emotion accompanied by tears. There may be sobbing or quiet weeping.

Facial Expression

1. Smiling is characterized by upturned corners of the mouth, brightening of the eyes, and a look of pleasure or contentment. Inexpressive refers to a neutral, at ease, relaxed, or blank look.
2. Sad is characterized by an unhappy, lonesome, sorrowful, or dejected look. There may be tears in the eyes.
3. Frightened is characterized by a look of fear, alarm, or heightened anxiety. Eyes appear wide open.
4. Frown is characterized by a downward turn of the corners of the mouth. Increased facial wrinkling in the forehead and around the mouth may appear.
5. Facial grimacing is characterized by a distorted, distressed look. The brow is more wrinkled as is the area around the mouth. Eyes may be squeezed shut.

Body Language

1. Relaxed is characterized by a calm, restful, mellow appearance. The person seems to be taking it easy.
2. Tense is characterized by a strained, apprehensive, or worried appearance. The jaw may be clenched (exclude any contractures).
3. Distressed pacing is characterized by activity that seems unsettled. There may be a fearful, worried, or disturbed element present. The rate may be faster or slower.

4. Fidgeting is characterized by restless movement. Squirming about or wiggling in the chair may occur. The person might be hitching a chair across the room. Repetitive touching, tugging, or rubbing body parts can also be observed.
5. Rigid is characterized by stiffening of the body. The arms and/or legs are tight and inflexible. The trunk may appear straight and unyielding (exclude any contractures).
6. Fists clenched is characterized by tightly closed hands. They may be opened and closed repeatedly or held tightly shut.
7. Knees pulled up is characterized by flexing the legs and drawing the knees up toward the chest. An overall troubled appearance (exclude any contractures).
8. Pulling or pushing away is characterized by resistiveness upon approach or to care. The person is trying to escape by yanking or wrenching him or herself free or shoving you away.
9. Striking out is characterized by hitting, kicking, grabbing, punching, biting, or other form of personal assault.

Consolability

1. No need to console is characterized by a sense of well being. The person appears content.
2. Distracted or reassured by voice or touch is characterized by a disruption in the behavior when the person is spoken to or touched. The behavior stops during the period of interaction with no indication that the person is at all distressed.
3. Unable to console, distract or reassure is characterized by the inability to sooth the person or stop a behavior with words or actions. No amount of comforting, verbal or physical, will alleviate the behavior.

Note. Reprinted from "Development and Psychometric Evaluation of the Pain Assessment in Advanced Dementia (PAINAD) Scale," (2003) by V. Warden, A. C. Hurley, and L. Volicer, *Journal of the American Medical Directors Association, 4*(1), pp. 9–15. Copyright 2003, with permission from American Medical Directors Association.

[a] Five-item observational tool (see the description of each item).

[b] Total scores range from 0 to 10 (based on a scale of 0 to 2 for five items), with a higher score indicating more severe pain (0 = no pain to 10 = severe pain).

- Sexuality among older adults is complicated by many issues:

  - Older adults may experience performance anxiety.
  - Older adults may not be familiar with the risks of sexually transmitted diseases and appropriate prevention.
  - Negative self-concepts and role changes that frequently occur in response to chronic illness may impact the experience of sexuality for older adults. The results might be

    - Fear of rejection or failure
    - Boredom
    - Hostility about sexual performance

  - Past sexual history such as delays in sexual development or sexual abuse may continue to impact sexuality in the later years.
  - Older adults tend to be reluctant to discuss sexual issues with health care providers.
  - Normal physiological changes among aging women:

    - A decrease in circulating estrogen, resulting in a thinning of the vaginal epithelium, the labia majora, and the subcutaneous tissue in the mons pubis.
    - The vaginal canal shortens and loses elasticity.
    - Follicular depletion of the ovaries as a result of a decrease in circulating estrogen, which leads to a further decline in the secretion of estrogen and progesterone.
    - Dyspareunia (painful intercourse) may result.
    - Orgasmic dysfunction and vaginismus may also result from the decrease in the amount of circulating estrogen and progesterone.

  - Normal physiological changes of aging men:

    - Viropause, andropause, or male menopause
    - Increased time needed to develop an erection and ejaculate
    - Erections may require direct penile stimulation

  - In both sexes, the physiological changes in hormone secretion affect four areas of sexual response:

    - Arousal
    - Orgasm
    - Postorgasm
    - Extragenital changes

  - Normal changes of aging may change or delay the sexual response of older adults; however, sexual dysfunction is not a normal process of aging.
  - Chronic illnesses such as depression and diabetes impact sexual function among older adults.
  - Medications that are commonly used among older adults can affect sexual function. These medications include

    - Antidepressants
    - Antihypertensives
    - Antipsychotics
    - Statin medications
    - H_2 blockers

- Surgery to prostate gland and breasts frequently interferes with the normal sexual function of older men and women.
- The loss of partners in older adulthood also significantly impacts sexuality.
- A sexual assessment is the first step needed to assess the sexuality of older adults (see chapter 8 for sexual assessment guidelines).

- Teaching regarding normal and pathological aging changes is needed.
- Interventions to promote sexuality among older adults may focus on

    - Promotion of erectile function among older men

        - Erectile agents such as sildenafil citrate (Viagra®), vardenafil hydrochloride (Levitra®), and tadalifil (Cilalis®) may aid in the treatment of erectile dysfunction among older men.
        - These medications are hazardous in men with history of heart failure, in patients with borderline hypotension, and with the use of nitrates.

    - The use of touch to create intimacy
    - Maintenance of privacy for sexual relationships
    - Consideration of client safety

        - Necessary equipment, such as grab bars
        - Condoms for safe sex

- For older adults with dementia, it is essential to conduct highly accurate assessments and document their ability to be involved in the decision-making process.
- Problematic sexual behaviors may occur in response to unmet sexual needs in older adults with dementia. These may include

    - Public masturbation
    - Exposure
    - Making sexually inappropriate comments
    - Sexual gestures

- Effective assessment and planning of care can help the older adult to meet their sexual needs in a dignified and respectful manner and will likely eliminate the behavior.

Elder Neglect and Abuse

- It is estimated that approximately one million cases of elder mistreatment occur annually.
- This number is likely an underestimation, because elder abuse is frequently not reported for several reasons.

    - Victims may fear retaliation.
    - Victims may feel shame.
    - Victims may have a desire or need to protect the abuser.
    - There is a lack of mandatory universal reporting laws.

11.1 Elder Assessment Instrument

I General Assessment	Very Good	Good	Poor	Very Poor	Unable to Assess
1. Clothing					
2. Hygiene					
3. Nutrition					
4. Skin integrity					
5. Additional Comments:					

II Possible Abuse Indicators	No Evidence	Possible Evidence	Probable Evidence	Definite Evidence	Unable to Assess
6. Bruising					
7. Lacerations					
8. Fractures					
9. Various stages of healing of any bruises or fractures					
10. Evidence of sexual abuse					
11. Statement by elder re: abuse					
12. Additional Comments:					

III Possible Neglect Indicators	No Evidence	Possible Evidence	Probable Evidence	Definite Evidence	Unable to Assess
13. Contractures					
14. Decubiti					
15. Dehydration					
16. Diarrhea					
17. Depression					
18. Impaction					
19. Malnutrition					
20. Urine burns					
21. Poor hygiene					
22. Failure to respond to warning of obvious disease					
23. Inappropriate medications (under/over)					
24. Repetitive hospital admissions due to probable failure of health care surveillance					
25. Statement by elder re: neglect					
26. Additional Comments:					

IV Possible Exploitation Indicators	No Evidence	Possible Evidence	Probable Evidence	Definite Evidence	Unable to Assess
27. Misuse of money					
28. Evidence of financial exploitation					
29. Reports of demands for goods in exchange for services					
30. Inability to account for money or property					
31. Statement by elder re: exploitation					
32. Additional Comments:					

V Possible Abandonment Indicators	No Evidence	Possible Evidence	Probable Evidence	Definite Evidence	Unable to Assess
33. Evidence that a caretaker has withdrawn care precipitously without alternate arrangements					
34. Evidence that elder is left alone in an unsafe environment for extended periods of time without adequate support					
35. Statement by elder re: abandonment					
36. Additional Comments:					

VI Summary	No Evidence	Possible Evidence	Probable Evidence	Definite Evidence	Unable to Assess
37. Evidence of abuse					
38. Evidence of neglect					
39. Evidence of exploitation					
40. Evidence of abandonment					
41. Additional Comments:					

VII   Comments and Follow-up

Note. Adapted from "Assessing Elder Abuse: A Study," by T. Fulmer and V. M. Cahill. 1984. *Journal of Gerontological Nursing. 10*(12), pp. 16–20; "Elder Abuse and Neglect Assessment." by T. Fulmer. 2003. *Journal of Gerontological Nursing. 29*(6), pp. 4–5. Reprinted from "Abuse of the Elderly: Screening and Detection." by T. Fulmer, S. Street, and K. Carr. 1984. *Journal of Emergency Nursing. 10*(3). pp. 131–140. Copyright 1984, with permission from The Emergency Nurses Association.

■ Elder abuse is difficult to assess (Exhibit 11.1), but red-flag symptoms include

  ■ Unexplained injuries or signs of neglect or mistreatment
  ■ Mismatch between an older adult's explanation of injury and his or her physical appearance
  ■ Conflicting stories between victim and caregiver
  ■ Caregiver refusal to leave victim alone

■ Types of abuse:

  ■ Physical abuse—inflicting physical injury or pain
  ■ Psychological abuse—infliction of mental anguish, such as threats, insults, and purposeful social isolation
  ■ Active neglect—purposeful withholding of necessities
  ■ Passive neglect—caregiver's inability to identify the older adult's needs or to perform the tasks essential to meet the older adult's needs
  ■ Sexual abuse—sexual assault or rape of an older adult
  ■ Financial abuse—exploiting the older adult's funds, property, or assets

■ Many older adults may exhibit characteristics of multiple types of mistreatment with a wide range of severity.
■ If elder abuse or neglect is suspected, the health care provider must report it immediately to the area ombudsman, whose job it is to act as a clearinghouse for complaints and problems, agency social service personnel, or the local adult protective services.

  ■ Document assessment effectively using photographs when possible.
  ■ Follow through to make sure the older adult is not returned to an unsafe situation.

References

American Geriatrics Society Panel on Chronic Pain in Older Persons. (1998). The management of chronic pain in older persons. *Journal of American Geriatric Society, 46,* 635–651.

Flaherty, E. (2007). *Try this: Pain assessment in older adults, 7.* Retrieved July 14, 2007, from http://www.hartfordign.org/publications/trythis/issue07.pdf

Fulmer, T., & V. M. Cahill (1984). Assessing elder abuse: A study. *Journal of Gerontological Nursing, 10*(12), 16–20.

Fulmer, T., Street, S., & Carr, K. (1984). Abuse of the elderly: Screening and detection. *Journal of Emergency Nursing, 10*(3), 131–140.

Lindau, S. T., Schumm, L. P., Laumann, E. O., Levinson, W., O'Muircheartaigh, C. A., & Waite, L. J. (2007). A study of sexuality and health among older adults in the United States. *The New England Journal of Medicine, 357,* 762–774.

Pediatric Pain Sourcebook. (2007). Faces pain scale. Retrieved March 23, 2008, from http://painsourcebook.ca/pdfs/pps92.pdf

Warden, V., Hurley, A. C., & Volicer, L. (2003). Development and psychometric evaluation of the Pain Assessment in Advanced Dementia (PAINAD) Scale. *Journal of the American Medical Directors Association, 4*(1), 9–15.

12

Organizational and Health Policy Issues

Advocacy for Older Adults

- Older adults as a group have taken action to prevent the effects of ageism on health care policy.
- Older adults have formed two large and influential national organizations that provide them with representation concerning legislative issues and resources for successful aging.
- American Association of Retired Persons (AARP)

    - AARP is the nation's leading and most powerful organization for people aged 50 and older.
    - The organization has substantial influence on policy making at the federal and state levels.
    - AARP has 36 million members—over 50% of older adults.
    - The membership is growing quickly, with a new member joining AARP every 11 seconds.
    - The name is misleading, because many members of AARP are not retired.

- AARP is a nonprofit, nonpartisan membership whose primary goal is to help older people live with independence, dignity, and purpose.
- An important component of the organization is its lobbying ability and influence on legislative issues of importance to older adults. With the assistance of AARP, the rights of older adults continue to be heard loudly on Capitol Hill.

- National Council on Aging (NCOA)

  - NCOA is a nonprofit organization that plays an influential role in providing information, technical assistance, and research in the field of aging.
  - It maintains a national information clearinghouse related to aging, plans conferences on aging issues, conducts research on aging, supports demonstration programs related to aging, and maintains a comprehensive library of materials associated with every aspect of aging.

Health Care Delivery Systems

- As a result of the vast improvements in health care technology, health care costs increased 12% to 14% per year in the 1970s and began to decrease slightly in the 1980s.
- Although the health care delivery system has improved vastly over the past century, many of the currently available interventions to detect disease early and treat disease effectively are not accessible to older adults because

  - Many older adults are uninsured.
  - Insurance might not cover a necessary test, procedure, or treatment.
  - Many older adults lack transportation to health care providers.
  - Primary providers of geriatric care are not widely available.

Reimbursement

- Reimbursement for health care has changed as a result of increasing costs. Allowable expenses under Medicare and Medicaid plans as well as private insurances have diminished in many cases and have been removed altogether in some cases.

  - The lack of reimbursement for medications and treatments for illness and the inability to pay out of pocket for these expensive treatments have resulted in an increase in the rates of noncompliance or nonadherence to medication regimes.
  - About half of all patients take the medications as prescribed upon leaving the physician's office. The other half take the medications incorrectly or not at all. One-third of those who take the medications incorrectly don't take them at all; one-third take some of the medications prescribed; and one-third do not even fill the prescription.

- Little, if any, time is spent on how to assist patients without health insurance to obtain needed health care.
- Regardless of the reason, many older adults need financial assistance to pay for health care.
- Often hospitals have programs to help older adults finance their health care over a period of months or to excuse the older adult from paying, if legitimately he or she cannot afford to do so.
- Physicians and other health care providers may offer the same payment alternatives for services received at private physicians' offices.
- Physicians in private practice may also have samples of medications to distribute to low-income older adults.
- Clinics often have sliding scales to make health care in these facilities more affordable. There are also various state-run programs that help older adults with resources for financing or finding health care that is affordable.

Older Americans Act

- Title III of the Older Americans Act of 1965 directed attention toward public and private health care systems to provide improved access to services and advocacy for older adults.
- This program improved community services such as home-delivered meals, transportation, home health care and homemaking assistance, adult day care, home repair, and legal assistance—all of which allow many older adults to remain functionally independent and community dwelling.
- These programs are administered within local area agencies on aging (AAA) in each state. AAAs provide older adults and health care providers with a resource with which to access and afford health care.
- To locate the area agency on aging in each state, use the links tab located at http://www.n4a.org. In addition to this Web resource, the administration on aging offers a toll-free Eldercare Locator telephone number—(800) 677-1116—to help older adults, families, and health care providers obtain necessary community services throughout the United States. Operators at Eldercare Locator assist callers to find information and assistance to address health care and other issues to ensure high functioning and quality of life.
- In addition to AAAs, senior service offices in hospitals are good sources of information about hospital and community-based resources.

Medicare and Medigap

- Medicare is a federal program that was enacted into law in 1965 during a time in U.S. history known as The Great Society. Medicare was among several programs that were started during this period with the specific aim of assisting the poor, the disabled, and older people to have a better quality of health care and quality of life.

- Older adults who have not paid into the U.S. Social Security system, either because they were never employed or because they immigrated to the United States as older adults must buy into the Medicare system to receive these benefits.
- The large majority of people age 65 and older are enrolled in Medicare.
- To be eligible to receive Medicare, older adults must have contributed to Social Security or the Medicare system during their working years or had a spouse who had worked and contributed to these systems.
- Medicare is paid for by the government and therefore involves regulation, including the need for institutions receiving Medicare reimbursement to complete full resident assessment instruments within 14 days and a plan of care within 21 days of facility admission.
- Health care delivery under Medicare is provided by private physicians, hospitals, nurses, nurse practitioners, and various health care facilities, not Medicare employees.
- Private physicians who treat Medicare patients receive 80% of the usual customary and reasonable (UCR) fee for services provided if they accept Medicare assignment. If they do not, they can charge no more than 115% of the amount allowed by Medicare, and the client must pay the 20% remaining UCR and any other amount up to 115%.
- Physicians are often hesitant to accept the low reimbursement for older adults through Medicare, and patients are hesitant to receive care from physicians who do not accept Medicare assignment because of the need to finance the co-pay. Consequently, there is a shortage of primary care physicians to treat the increasing health care needs of older adults.
- Medicare has two parts.

  - Part A provides hospital insurance for older adults. In the event that an older adult requires hospitalization, this is the type of Medicare insurance that would pay for the hospital stay. In addition, this is the portion of Medicare that pays for short-term nursing home or home care visits after hospitalization in order for the older adult to return to prehospitalization health status. Medicare Part A also pays for hospice care (which is discussed in chapter 7). Generally, there is no premium for this insurance. In other words, if older adults meet the eligibility for Medicare as stated above, they are automatically enrolled in the Part A Medicare plan.
  - Part B pays for visits to physicians, nurse practitioners, and for other health care expenditures, such as X-rays, physical and occupational outpatient therapy, and laboratory tests. There is a monthly premium that older adults must pay for this type of Medicare plan. The current monthly premium is about $78. The amount is usually deducted from the recipient's monthly social security checks. Part B Medicare also requires recipients to pay the first $110 of charges before it will begin reimbursement. This is known as a deductible. The deductible for Part B Medicare is likely to increase annually. Coverage of Medicare for health care needs of older adults is detailed in Table 12.1.

12.1 Medicare Coverage for the Health Care Needs of Older Adults

Service or Supply	What is covered, and when?
Acupuncture	Medicare doesn't cover acupuncture.
Ambulance Services	Medicare covers limited ambulance services. If you need to go to a hospital or skilled nursing facility (SNF). ambulance services are covered only if transportation in any other vehicle would endanger your health. Medicare helps pay for necessary ambulance transportation to the closest appropriate facility that can provide the care you need. If you choose to go to another facility farther away, Medicare payment is based on how much it would cost to go to the closest appropriate facility. All ambulance suppliers must accept assignment. Medicare generally doesn't pay for ambulance transportation to a doctor's office. Air ambulance is paid only in the most severe situations. If you could have gone by land ambulance without serious danger to your life or health. Medicare pays only the land ambulance rate, and you are responsible for the difference.
Ambulatory Surgical Centers	Medicare covers services given in an Ambulatory Surgical Center for a covered surgical procedure.
Anesthesia	Medicare covers anesthesia services along with medical and surgical benefits. Medicare Part A covers anesthesia you get while in an inpatient hospital. Medicare Part B covers anesthesia you get as an outpatient.
Artificial Limbs and Eyes	Medicare helps pay for artificial limbs and eyes. For more information. see Prosthetic Devices.
Blood	Medicare doesn't cover the first three pints of blood you get under Part A and Part B combined in a calendar year. Part A covers blood you get as an inpatient, and Part B covers blood you get as an outpatient and in a freestanding Ambulatory Surgical Center.
Bone Mass Measurement	Medicare covers bone mass measurements ordered by a doctor or qualified practitioner who is treating you if you meet one or more of the following conditions: Women ■ You are being treated for low estrogen levels and are at clinical risk for osteoporosis, based on your medical history and other findings.

(continued)

12.1 Medicare Coverage for the Health Care Needs of Older Adults (*continued*)

Service or Supply	What is covered, and when?
	Men and Women
	■ Your X-rays show possible osteoporosis, osteopenia, or vertebrae fractures.
	■ You are on prednisone or steroid-type drugs or are planning to begin such treatment.
	■ You have been diagnosed with primary hyperparathyroidism.
	■ You are being monitored to see if your osteoporosis drug therapy is working.
	The test is covered once every two years for qualified individuals and more often if medically necessary.
Braces (arm, leg, back, and neck)	Medicare covers arm, leg, back, and neck braces. For more information, see Orthotics.
Breast Prostheses	Medicare covers breast prostheses (including a surgical brassiere) after a mastectomy. For more information, see Prosthetic Devices.
Canes/Crutches	Medicare covers canes and crutches. Medicare doesn't cover canes for the blind. For more information, see Durable Medical Equipment.
Cardiac Rehabilitation Programs	Medicare covers comprehensive programs that include exercise, education, and counseling for patients whose doctor referred them and who have 1) had a heart attack in the last 12 months, 2) had coronary bypass surgery, 3) stable angina pectoris, 4) had heart valve repair/replacement, 5) had angioplasty or coronary stenting, and/or 6) had a heart or heart-lung transplant. These programs may be given by the outpatient department of a hospital or in doctor-directed clinics.
Cardiovascular Screening	Medicare covers screening tests for cholesterol, lipid, and triglyceride levels every five years. Ask your doctor to test your cholesterol, lipid, and triglyceride levels so he or she can help you prevent a heart attack or stroke.
Chemotherapy	Medicare covers chemotherapy for patients who are hospital inpatients, outpatients, or patients in a doctor's office or freestanding clinics. In the inpatient hospital setting, Part A covers chemotherapy. In a hospital outpatient setting, freestanding facility, or doctor's office, Part B covers chemotherapy.

Chiropractic Services	Medicare covers manipulation of the spine if medically necessary to correct a subluxation (when one or more of the bones of your spine moves out of position) when provided by chiropractors or other qualified providers.
Clinical Trials	Medicare covers routine costs, like doctor visits and tests, if you take part in a qualifying clinical trial. Clinical trials test new types of medical care, like how well a new cancer drug works. Clinical trials help doctors and researchers see if the new care works and if it is safe. Medicare doesn't pay for the experimental item being investigated, in most cases.
Colorectal Cancer Screening	Medicare covers several colorectal cancer screening tests. Talk with your doctor about the screening test that is right for you. All people age 50 and older with Medicare are covered. However, there is no minimum age for having a colonoscopy. Colonoscopy: Medicare covers this test once every 24 months if you are at high risk for colorectal cancer. If you aren't at high risk for colorectal cancer, the test is covered once every 120 months, but not sooner than 48 months after a screening sigmoidoscopy. Fecal Occult Blood Test: Medicare covers this lab test once every 12 months. Flexible Sigmoidoscopy: Medicare covers this test once every 48 months for people 50 and older. Barium Enema: Once every 48 months (high risk every 24 months) when used instead of a flexible sigmoidoscopy or colonoscopy.
Commode Chairs	Medicare covers commode chairs that your doctor orders for use in your home if you are confined to your bedroom. For more information, see Durable Medical Equipment on page 46.
Cosmetic Surgery	Medicare generally doesn't cover cosmetic surgery unless it is needed because of accidental injury or to improve the function of a malformed part of the body. Medicare covers breast reconstruction if you had a mastectomy because of breast cancer.
Custodial Care (help with activities of daily living, like bathing, dressing, using the bathroom, and eating)	Medicare doesn't cover custodial care when it's the only kind of care you need. Care is considered custodial when it's for the purpose of helping you with activities of daily living or personal needs that could be done safely and reasonably by people without professional skills or training. For example, custodial care includes help getting in and out of bed, bathing, dressing, eating, and taking medicine.
Dental Services	Medicare doesn't cover routine dental care or most dental procedures such as cleanings, fillings, tooth extractions, or dentures. Medicare doesn't pay for dental plates or other dental devices. Medicare Part A will pay for certain dental services that you get when you are in the hospital. Medicare Part A can pay for hospital stays if you need to have emergency or complicated dental procedures, even when the dental care itself isn't covered.

(continued)

12.1 Medicare Coverage for the Health Care Needs of Older Adults (*continued*)

Service or Supply	What is covered, and when?
Diabetes Screening	Medicare covers tests to check for diabetes. These tests are available if you have any of the following risk factors: high blood pressure, dyslipidemia (history of abnormal cholesterol and triglyceride levels), obesity, or a history of high blood sugar. Medicare also covers these tests if you have two or more of the following characteristics: ■ age 65 or older. ■ overweight. ■ family history of diabetes (parents, brothers, sisters). ■ a history of gestational diabetes (diabetes during pregnancy) or delivery of a baby weighing more than 9 pounds. Based on the results of these tests, you may be eligible for up to two diabetes screenings every year.
Diabetes Supplies and Services	Medicare covers some diabetes supplies, including ■ blood glucose test strips. ■ blood glucose monitor. ■ lancet devices and lancets. and ■ glucose control solutions for checking the accuracy of test strips and monitors. There may be limits on how much or how often you get these supplies. For more information, see Durable Medical Equipment on page 149. Here are some ways you can make sure your Medicare diabetes medical supplies are covered: ■ Only accept supplies you have ordered. Medicare won't pay for supplies you didn't order. ■ Make sure you request your supply refills. Medicare won't pay for supplies sent from the supplier to you automatically. ■ All Medicare-enrolled pharmacies and suppliers must submit claims for glucose test strips. You can't send in the claim yourself. Medicare doesn't cover insulin (unless used with an insulin pump). insulin pens, syringes, needles. alcohol swabs, gauze. eye exams for glasses, and routine or yearly physical exams. If you use an external insulin pump. insulin and the pump could be covered as durable medical equipment. There may be some limits on covered supplies or how often you get them. Insulin and certain medical supplies used to inject insulin are covered under Medicare prescription drug coverage.

Therapeutic Shoes or Inserts: Medicare covers therapeutic shoes or inserts for people with diabetes who have severe diabetic foot disease. The doctor who treats your diabetes must certify your need for therapeutic shoes or inserts. The shoes and inserts must be prescribed by a podiatrist or other qualified doctor and provided by a podiatrist, orthotist, prosthetist, or pedorthist. Medicare helps pay for one pair of therapeutic shoes and inserts per calendar year. Shoe modifications may be substituted for inserts. The fitting of the shoes or inserts is covered in the Medicare payment for the shoes.

Medicare covers these diabetes services:

■ Diabetes Self-Management Training: Diabetes outpatient self-management training is a covered program to teach you to manage your diabetes. It includes education about self-monitoring of blood glucose, diet, exercise, and insulin.

If you've been diagnosed with diabetes, Medicare may cover up to 10 hours of initial diabetes self-management training. You may also qualify for up to two hours of follow-up training each year if

  ▪ it is provided in a group of 2 to 20 people.

  ▪ it lasts for at least 30 minutes.

  ▪ it takes place in a calendar year following the year you got your initial training, and

  ▪ your doctor or a qualified non-physician practitioner ordered it as part of your plan of care.

  ▪ Some exceptions apply if no group session is available or if your doctors or qualified non-physician practitioner says you have special needs that prevent you from participating in group training.

■ Yearly Eye Exam: Medicare covers yearly eye exams for diabetic retinopathy.

■ Foot Exam: A foot exam is covered every 6 months for people with diabetic peripheral neuropathy and loss of protective sensations, as long as you haven't seen a foot care professional for another reason between visits.

■ Glaucoma Screening: Medicare covers glaucoma screening every 12 months for people with diabetes or a family history of glaucoma, African Americans age 50 and older, or Hispanics age 65 and older.

■ Medical Nutrition Therapy Services: Medical nutrition therapy services are also covered for people with diabetes or kidney disease when referred by a doctor. These services can be given by a registered dietitian or Medicare-approved nutrition professional and include a nutritional assessment and counseling to help you manage your diabetes or kidney disease.

For more information, call 1-800-MEDICARE (1-800-633-4227). TTY users should call 1-877-486-2048.

(continued)

12.1 Medicare Coverage for the Health Care Needs of Older Adults (*continued*)

Service or Supply	What is covered, and when?
Diagnostic Tests, X-rays, and Lab Services	Medicare covers diagnostic tests like CT scans, MRIs, EKGs, and X-rays. Medicare also covers clinical diagnostic tests and lab services provided by certified laboratories enrolled in Medicare. Diagnostic tests and lab services are done to help your doctor diagnose or rule out a suspected illness or condition. Medicare doesn't cover most routine screening tests, like checking your hearing. Some preventive tests and screenings are covered by Medicare to help prevent, find, or manage a medical problem. For more information, see Preventive Services.
Dialysis (Kidney)	Medicare covers some kidney dialysis services and supplies, including the following: ■ Inpatient dialysis treatments (if you are admitted to a hospital for special care). ■ Outpatient maintenance dialysis treatments (when you get treatments in any Medicare-approved dialysis facility). ■ Certain home dialysis support services (may include visits by trained dialysis workers to check on your home dialysis, to help in dialysis emergencies when needed, and check your dialysis equipment and hemodialysis water supply). ■ Certain drugs for home dialysis, including heparin, the antidote for heparin when medically necessary, and topical anesthetics. ■ Erythropoiesis-stimulating agents (such as Epogen®, Epoetin alfa), or Darbepoetin alfa (Aranesp®) are drugs used to treat anemia if you have end-stage renal disease. For more information, see Prescription Drugs. ■ Self-dialysis training (includes training for you and the person helping you with your home dialysis treatments). ■ Home dialysis equipment and supplies (like alcohol, wipes, sterile drapes, rubber gloves, and scissors).
Doctor's Office Visits	Medicare covers medically necessary services you get from your doctor in his or her office, in a hospital, in a skilled nursing facility, in your home, or any other location. Routine annual physicals aren't covered, except the one-time "Welcome to Medicare" physical exam. Some preventive tests and screenings are covered by Medicare. See Preventive Services, and Pap Test/Pelvic Exam.
Drugs	See Prescription Drugs (Outpatient).

Durable Medical Equipment (DME)	Medicare covers Durable Medical Equipment (DME) that your doctor prescribes for use in your home. Only your own doctor can prescribe medical equipment for you.

Durable Medical Equipment is

▣ (long lasting) durable.

▣ used for a medical reason.

▣ not usually useful to someone who isn't sick or injured. and

▣ used in your home.

The Durable Medical Equipment that Medicare covers includes, but isn't limited to the following:

▣ Air-fluidized beds

▣ Blood glucose monitors

▣ Canes (canes for the blind aren't covered)

▣ Commode chairs

▣ Crutches

▣ Dialysis machines

▣ Home oxygen equipment and supplies

▣ Hospital beds

▣ Infusion pumps (and some medicines used in infusion pumps if considered reasonable and necessary)

▣ Nebulizers (and some medicines used in nebulizers if considered reasonable and necessary)

▣ Patient lifts (to lift patient from bed or wheelchair by hydraulic operation)

▣ Suction pumps

▣ Traction equipment

▣ Walkers

▣ Wheelchairs

Make sure your supplier is enrolled in Medicare and has a Medicare supplier number. Suppliers have to meet strict standards to qualify for a Medicare supplier number. Medicare won't pay your claim if your supplier doesn't have one. even if your supplier is a large chain or department store that sells more than just durable medical equipment.

(continued)

12.1 Medicare Coverage for the Health Care Needs of Older Adults (*continued*)

Service or Supply	What is covered, and when?
Emergency Room Services	Medicare covers emergency room services. Emergency services aren't covered in foreign countries, except in some instances in Canada and Mexico. For more information, see Travel.
	A medical emergency is when you believe that your health is in serious danger. You may have an injury or illness that requires immediate medical attention to prevent a severe disability or death.
	When you go to an emergency room, you will pay a copayment for each hospital service, and you will also pay coinsurance for each doctor who treats you.
	Note: If you are admitted to the hospital within three days of the emergency room visit for the same condition, the emergency room visit is included in the inpatient hospital care charges, not charged separately.
Equipment	See Durable Medical Equipment.
Eye Exams	Medicare doesn't cover routine eye exams.
	Medicare covers some preventive eye tests and screenings:
	■ See yearly eye exams under Diabetes Supplies and Services on page 25.
	■ See Glaucoma Screening.
	■ See Macular Degeneration.
Eyeglasses/Contact Lenses	Generally, Medicare doesn't cover eyeglasses or contact lenses.
	However, following cataract surgery with an implanted intraocular lens, Medicare helps pay for corrective lenses (spectacles or contact lenses) provided by a licensed and Medicare-approved opthalmologist. Services provided by a licensed and Medicare-approved opthalmologist may be covered, if they are authorized to provide this service in your state.
	Important:
	■ Only standard frames are covered.
	■ Lenses are covered even if you had the surgery before you had Medicare.
	■ Payment may be made for lenses for both eyes even though cataract surgery involved only one eye.

Eye Refractions	Medicare doesn't cover eye refractions.
Flu Shots	Medicare covers one flu shot per flu season. You can get a flu shot in the winter and the fall flu season of the same calendar year. All people with Medicare are covered.
Foot Care	Medicare generally doesn't cover routine foot care. Medicare Part B covers the services of a podiatrist (foot doctor) for medically necessary treatment of injuries or diseases of the foot (such as hammer toe, bunion deformities, and heel spurs). See Therapeutic Shoes and Foot Exam under Diabetes Supplies and Services starting.
Glaucoma Screening	Medicare covers glaucoma screening once every 12 months for people at high risk for glaucoma. This includes people with diabetes, a family history of glaucoma, African Americans age 50 and older, or Hispanic Americans age 65 and older. The screening must be done or supervised by an eye doctor who is legally allowed to do this service in your state.
Health Education/ Wellness Programs	Medicare generally doesn't cover health education and wellness programs. However, Medicare does cover medical nutrition therapy for some people and diabetes education for people with diabetes.
Hearing Exams/Hearing Aids	Medicare doesn't cover routine hearing exams, hearing aids, or exams for fitting hearing aids. In some cases, Medicare covers diagnostic hearing exams.
Hepatitis B Shots	Medicare covers this preventive service (three shots) for people at high or medium (intermediate) to high risk for Hepatitis B. Your risk for Hepatitis B increases if you have hemophilia, end-stage renal disease (permanent kidney failure requiring dialysis or a kidney transplant), or a condition that lowers your resistance to infection. Other factors may also increase your risk for Hepatitis B. Check with your doctor to see if you are at high to medium risk for Hepatitis B.
Home Health Care	Medicare covers some home health care if the following conditions are met: 1. Your doctor decides you need medical care in your home and makes a plan for your care at home, and 2. You need reasonable and necessary part-time or intermittent skilled nursing care and home health aide services, and physical therapy, occupational therapy, and speech-language pathology ordered by your doctor and provided by a Medicare-certified home health agency. This includes medical social services, other services, durable medical equipment (such as wheelchairs, hospital beds, oxygen, and walkers), and medical supplies for use at home. 3. You are homebound. This means you are normally unable to leave home and that leaving home is a major effort. When you leave home, it must be infrequent, for a short time. You may attend religious services. You may leave the house to get medical treatment, including therapeutic or psychosocial care. You can also get care in an adult day care program that is licensed or certified by your state or accredited to furnish adult day care services in your state, and 4. The home health agency caring for you must be approved by Medicare.

(continued)

Service or Supply	What is covered, and when?
	Medicare covers durable medical equipment (such as wheelchairs, hospital beds, oxygen, and walkers).
	Note for Women with Osteoporosis: Medicare helps pay for an injectable drug for osteoporosis in women who have Medicare Part B, meet the criteria for the Medicare home health benefit, and have a bone fracture that a doctor certifies was related to post-menopausal osteoporosis. You must also be certified by a doctor as unable to learn or unable to give yourself the drug by injection, and that family and/or caregivers are unable or unwilling to give the drug by injection.
	Medicare covers the visit by a home health nurse to give the drug.
Hospice Care	Medicare covers hospice care if
	▪ you are eligible for Medicare Part A.
	▪ your doctor and the hospice medical director certify that you are terminally ill and probably have less than six months to live.
	▪ you accept palliative (care to comfort) instead of care to cure your illness.
	▪ you sign a statement choosing hospice care instead of routine Medicare-covered benefits for your terminal illness, and
	▪ you get care from a Medicare-approved hospice program.
	Medicare allows a nurse practitioner to serve as an attending doctor for a patient who elects the hospice benefit. Nurse practitioners are prohibited from certifying a terminal diagnosis.
	Respite Care: Medicare also covers respite care if you are getting covered hospice care. Respite care is inpatient care given to a hospice patient so that the usual caregiver can rest. You can stay in a Medicare-approved facility, such as a hospice facility, hospital or nursing home, up to five days each time you get respite care.
	Medicare will still pay for covered services for any health problems that aren't related to your terminal illness.
Hospital Bed	See Durable Medical Equipment.

Hospital Care (Inpatient) for Outpatient Services.	Medicare covers inpatient hospital care when all of the following are true: ■ A doctor says you need inpatient hospital care to treat your illness or injury. ■ You need the kind of care that can be given only in a hospital. ■ The hospital is enrolled in Medicare. ■ The Utilization Review Committee of the hospital approves your stay while you are in the hospital. ■ A Quality Improvement Organization approves your stay after the bill is submitted. Medicare-covered hospital services include the following: a semiprivate room, meals, general nursing, and other hospital services and supplies. This includes care you get in critical access hospitals and inpatient mental health care. This doesn't include private-duty nursing, a television, or telephone in your room. It also doesn't include a private room, unless medically necessary.
Implantable Cardiac Defibrillator	Medicare covers defibrillators for many people diagnosed with congestive heart failure.
Kidney (Dialysis)	See Dialysis.
Lab Services	Medicare covers medically necessary diagnostic lab services that are ordered by your treating doctor when they are provided by a Clinical Laboratory Improvement Amendments (CLIA)–certified laboratory enrolled in Medicare. For more information, see Diagnostic Tests.
Macular Degeneration	Medicare covers certain treatments for some patients with age-related macular degeneration (AMD) like ocular photodynamic therapy with verteporfin (Visudyne®).
Mammogram (Screening)	Medicare covers a screening mammogram once every 12 months (11 full months must have gone by from the last screening) for all women with Medicare age 40 and older. You can also get one baseline mammogram between ages 35 and 39.
Mental Health Care	Medicare covers mental health care given by a doctor or a qualified mental health professional. Before you get treatment, ask your doctor, psychologist, social worker, or other health professional if they accept Medicare payment. Inpatient Mental Health Care: Medicare covers inpatient mental health care services. These services can be given in psychiatric units of a general hospital or in a specialty psychiatric hospital that cares for people with mental health problems. Medicare helps pay for inpatient mental health services in the same way that it pays for all other inpatient hospital care. Note: If you are in a specialty psychiatric hospital, Medicare only helps for a total of 190 days of inpatient care during your lifetime.

(continued)

12.1 Medicare Coverage for the Health Care Needs of Older Adults (*continued*)

Service or Supply	What is covered, and when?
	Outpatient Mental Health Care: Medicare covers mental health services on an outpatient basis by either a doctor, clinical psychologist, clinical social worker, clinical nurse specialist, or physician assistant in an office setting, clinic, or hospital outpatient department.
	Partial Hospitalization: Partial hospitalization may be available for you. It is a structured program of active psychiatric treatment that is more intense than the care you get in your doctor or therapist's office. For Medicare to cover a partial hospitalization program, a doctor must say that you would otherwise need inpatient treatment.
	Medicare covers the services of specially qualified non-physician practitioners such as clinical psychologists, clinical social workers, nurse practitioners, clinical nurse specialists, and physician assistants, as allowed by state and local law for medically necessary services.
Nursing Home Care	Most nursing home care is custodial care. Generally, Medicare doesn't cover custodial care. Medicare Part A only covers skilled nursing care given in a certified skilled nursing facility (SNF) or in your home (if you are homebound) if medically necessary, but not custodial care (such as helping with bathing or dressing).
Nutrition Therapy Services (Medical)	Medicare covers medical nutrition therapy services, when ordered by a doctor, for people with kidney disease (but who aren't on dialysis) or who have a kidney transplant, or people with diabetes. These services can be given by a registered dietitian or Medicare-approved nutrition professional and include nutritional assessment, one-on-one counseling, and therapy through an interactive telecommunications system. See Diabetes Supplies and Services.
Occupational Therapy	See Physical Therapy/Occupational Therapy/Speech–Language Pathology.
Orthotics	Medicare covers artificial limbs and eyes, and arm, leg, back and neck braces. Medicare doesn't pay for orthopedic shoes unless they are a necessary part of the leg brace. Medicare doesn't pay for dental plates or other dental devices. See Diabetes Supplies and Services (Therapeutic Shoes).

Ostomy Supplies	Medicare covers ostomy supplies for people who have had a colostomy, ileostomy, or urinary ostomy. Medicare covers the amount of supplies your doctor says you need, based on your condition.
Outpatient Hospital Services	Medicare covers medically necessary services you get as an outpatient from a Medicare-participating hospital for diagnosis or treatment of an illness or injury. Covered outpatient hospital services include
	▪ services in an emergency room or outpatient clinic, including same-day surgery.
	▪ laboratory tests billed by the hospital.
	▪ mental health care in a partial hospitalization program, if a doctor certifies that inpatient treatment would be required without it.
	▪ X-rays and other radiology services billed by the hospitals.
	▪ medical supplies such as splints and casts.
	▪ screenings and preventive services, and
	▪ certain drugs and biologicals that you can't give yourself.
Oxygen Therapy	Medicare covers the rental of oxygen equipment. Or, if you own your own equipment, Medicare will help pay for oxygen contents and supplies for the delivery of oxygen when all of these conditions are met:
	▪ Your doctor says you have a severe lung disease or you're not getting enough oxygen and your condition might improve with oxygen therapy.
	▪ Your arterial blood gas level falls within a certain range.
	▪ Other alternative measures have failed.
	Under the above conditions Medicare helps pay for
	▪ systems for furnishing oxygen.
	▪ containers that store oxygen.
	▪ tubing and related supplies for the delivery of oxygen, and
	▪ oxygen contents.
	If oxygen is provided only for use during sleep, portable oxygen wouldn't be covered. Portable oxygen isn't covered when provided only as a backup to a stationary oxygen system.
Pap Test/Pelvic Exam	Medicare covers Pap tests and pelvic exams (and a clinical breast exam) for all women once every 24 months. Medicare covers this test and exam once every 12 months if you are at high risk for cervical or vaginal cancer or if you are of childbearing age and have had an abnormal Pap test in the past 36 months. If you have your Pap test, pelvic exam, and clinical breast exam on the same visit as a routine physical exam, you pay for the physical exam. Routine physical exams aren't covered by Medicare, except for the one-time "Welcome to Medicare" physical exam.

(continued)

12.1 Medicare Coverage for the Health Care Needs of Older Adults (*continued*)

Service or Supply	What is covered, and when?
Physical Exams (routine) ("One-time Welcome to Medicare" physical exam)	Routine physical exams aren't generally covered by Medicare. Medicare covers a one-time review of your health, as well as education and counseling about the preventive services you need, including certain screenings and shots. Referrals for other care, if you need them, will also be covered. *Important:* You must have the physical exam within the first six months you have Medicare Part B (deductibles and coinsurance apply).
Physical Therapy/ Occupational Therapy/ Speech-Language Pathology	Medicare helps pay for medically necessary outpatient physical and occupational therapy and speech-language pathology services when ■ your doctor or therapist sets up the plan of treatment, and ■ your doctor periodically reviews the plan to see how long you will need therapy. You can get outpatient services from a Medicare-approved outpatient provider such as a participating hospital or skilled nursing facility, or from a participating home health agency, rehabilitation agency, or a comprehensive outpatient rehabilitation facility. Also, you can get services from a Medicare-approved physical or occupational therapist, in private practice, in his or her office, or in your home. (Medicare doesn't pay for services given by a speech-language pathologist in private practice.) In 2007, there may be limits on physical therapy, occupational therapy, and speech-language pathology services. If so, there may be exceptions to these limits.
Pneumococcal Shot	Medicare covers the pneumococcal shot to help prevent pneumococcal infections. Most people only need this preventive shot once in their lifetime. Talk with your doctor to see if you need this shot.
Prescription Drugs (Outpatient) Very Limited Coverage	Part B covers a limited number of outpatient prescription drugs. Your pharmacy or doctor must accept assignment on Medicare-covered prescription drugs. Part B covers drugs that aren't usually self-administered when you are given them in a hospital outpatient department. You can get comprehensive drug coverage by joining a Medicare drug plan (also called "Part D"). For more information. The following outpatient prescription drugs are covered: ■ Some Antigens: Medicare will help pay for antigens if they are prepared by a doctor and given by a properly instructed person (who could be the patient) under doctor supervision. ■ Osteoporosis Drugs: Medicare helps pay for an injectable drug for osteoporosis for certain women with Medicare. See note for women with osteoporosis, under Home Health Care. ■ Erythropoisis–stimulating agents (such as Epogen.® Epoetin alfa, or Darbepoetin alfa Aranesp®): Medicare will help pay for erythropoietin by injection if you have end-stage renal disease (permanent kidney failure) and need this drug to treat anemia.

■ Blood Clotting Factors: If you have hemophilia, Medicare will help pay for clotting factors you give yourself by injection.

■ Injectable Drugs: Medicare covers most injectable drugs given by a licensed medical practitioner, if the drug is considered reasonable and necessary for treatment.

■ Immunosuppressive Drugs: Medicare covers immunosuppressive drug therapy for transplant patients if the transplant was paid for by Medicare (or paid by private insurance that paid as a primary payer to your Medicare Part A coverage) in a Medicare-certified facility.

■ Oral Cancer Drugs: Medicare will help pay for some cancer drugs you take by mouth if the same drug is available in injectable form.

Currently, Medicare covers the following cancer drugs you take by mouth:

■ Capecitabine (brand name Xeloda®)

■ Cyclophosphamide (brand name Cytoxan®)

■ Methotrexate

■ Temozolomide (brand name Temodar®)

■ Busulfan (brand name Myleran®)

■ Etoposide (brand name VePesid®)

■ Melphalan (brand name Alkeran®)

As new cancer drugs become available, Medicare may cover them.

■ Oral Anti-Nausea Drugs: Medicare will help pay for oral anti-nausea drugs used as part of an anti-cancer chemotherapeutic regimen. The drugs must be administered within 48 hours and must be used as a full therapeutic replacement for the intravenous anti-nausea drugs that would otherwise be given.

Medicare also covers some drugs used in infusion pumps and nebulizers if considered reasonable and necessary.

Preventive Services

Medicare covers the following preventive services:

■ Bone Mass Measurement.

■ Cardiovascular Screening Blood Tests.

■ Colorectal Cancer Screening.

■ Diabetes Screenings.

■ Glaucoma Screening.

■ Mammogram Screening.

■ Nutrition Therapy Services.

(continued)

157

12.1 Medicare Coverage for the Health Care Needs of Older Adults (*continued*)

Service or Supply	What is covered, and when?
	■ Pap Test/Pelvic Exam. ■ Prostate Cancer Screening. ■ Shots on page 52 including - flu shot. - pneumococcal shot, and - Hepatitis B shot. ■ Smoking Cessation Counseling. ■ One-time "Welcome to Medicare" physical exam.
Prostate Cancer Screening	Medicare covers prostate screening tests once every 12 months for all men age 50 and older with Medicare (coverage begins the day after your 50th birthday). Covered tests include the following: ■ Digital Rectal Examination ■ Prostate Specific Antigen (PSA) Test
Prosthetic Devices	Medicare covers prosthetic devices needed to replace an internal body part or function. These include Medicare-approved corrective lenses needed after a cataract operation (see Eyeglasses/Contact Lenses), ostomy bags and certain related supplies (see Ostomy Supplies), and breast prostheses (including a surgical brassiere) after a mastectomy (see Breast Prostheses).
Radiation Therapy	Medicare covers radiation therapy for patients who are hospital inpatients or outpatients or patients in freestanding clinics.
Religious Nonmedical Health Care Institution (RNHCI)	Medicare doesn't cover the religious portion of RNHCI care. Medicare covers inpatient nonmedical care when the following conditions are met: ■ The RNHCI has agreed and is currently certified to participate in Medicare, and the Utilization Review Committee agrees that you'd require hospital or skilled nursing facility care if it weren't for your religious beliefs.

	You have a written agreement with Medicare indicating that your need for this form of care is based on your religious beliefs. The agreement must also indicate that if you decide to accept standard medical care you may have to wait longer to get RNHCI services in the future. You're always able to access medically necessary Medicare Part A services.
	The care provided is reasonable and necessary.
Respite Care	Medicare covers respite care for hospice patients (see Hospice Care).
Second Surgical Opinions	Medicare covers a second opinion before surgery that isn't an emergency. A second opinion is when another doctor gives his or her view about your health problem and how it should be treated. Medicare will also help pay for a third opinion if the first and second opinions are different.
Shots (Vaccinations)	Medicare covers the following shots: Flu Shot: Once per flu season. You can get a flu shot in the fall and the winter flu seasons of the same year. Hepatitis B Shot: Certain people with Medicare at medium to high risk for Hepatitis B. Pneumococcal Shot: One shot may be all you ever need. Ask your doctor.
Skilled Nursing Facility (SNF) Care	Medicare covers skilled care in a skilled nursing facility (SNF) under certain conditions for a limited time. Skilled care is health care given when you need skilled nursing or rehabilitation staff to manage, observe, and evaluate your care. Examples of skilled care include changing sterile dressings and physical therapy. Care that can be given by non-professional staff isn't considered skilled care. Medicare covers certain skilled care services that are needed daily on a short-term basis (up to 100 days). Medicare will cover skilled care if all these conditions are met: 1. You have Medicare Part A (Hospital Insurance) and have days left in your benefit period to use. 2. You have a qualifying hospital stay. This means an inpatient hospital stay of three consecutive days or more, including the day you're admitted to the hospital, but not including the day you leave the hospital. You must enter the SNF within a short time (generally 30 days) of leaving the hospital and require skilled services related to your hospital stay (see item 5). After you leave the SNF, if you reenter the same or another SNF within 30 days, you don't need another three-day qualifying hospital stay to get additional SNF benefits. This is also true if you stop getting skilled care while in the SNF and then start getting skilled care again within 30 days. 3. Your doctor has decided that you need daily skilled care. It must be given by, or under the direct supervision of, skilled nursing or rehabilitation staff. If you are in the SNF for skilled rehabilitation services only, your care is considered daily care even if these therapy services are offered just five or six days a week, as long as you need and get the therapy services each day they are offered.

(continued)

12.1 Medicare Coverage for the Health Care Needs of Older Adults (*continued*)

Service or Supply	What is covered, and when?
	4. You get these skilled services in a SNF that is certified by Medicare.
	5. You need these skilled services for a medical condition that
	▪ was treated during a qualifying three-day hospital stay, or
	▪ started while you were getting care in the SNF for a medical condition that was treated during a qualifying three-day hospital stay. For example, if you are in the SNF because you had a stroke, and you develop an infection that requires I.V. antibiotics and you meet the conditions listed in items 1–4, Medicare will cover skilled care.
Smoking Cessation (Counseling to stop smoking)	Medicare covers minimal regular doctor's office visits, and up to 8 face-to-face visits in a 12-month period if you are diagnosed with an illness caused or complicated by tobacco use, or you take a medicine that is affected by tobacco.
Speech-Language Pathology	See Physical Therapy/Occupational Therapy/Speech-Language Pathology.
Substance-Related Disorders	Medicare covers treatment for substance-related disorders in inpatient or outpatient settings. Certain limits apply.
Supplies (you use at home)	Medicare generally doesn't cover common medical supplies like bandages and gauze. Supplies furnished as part of a doctor's service are covered by Medicare, and payment is included in Medicare's doctor payment. Doctors don't bill for supplies.
	Medicare covers some diabetes and dialysis supplies. See Diabetes Supplies and Services on page 146 and Dialysis (Kidney).
	For items such as walkers, oxygen, and wheelchairs, see Durable Medical Equipment.
Surgical Dressings	Medicare covers surgical dressings when medically necessary for the treatment of a surgical or surgically treated wound.
Therapeutic Shoes	See Diabetes Supplies and Services (Therapeutic Shoes).

Transplants (Doctor Services)	Medicare covers doctor services for transplants, see Transplants (Facility Charges).
Transplants (Facility Charges)	Medicare covers transplants of the heart, lung, kidney, pancreas, intestine/multivisceral, bone marrow, cornea, and liver under certain conditions and, for some types of transplants, only at Medicare-approved facilities. Medicare only approves facilities for kidney, heart, liver, lung, intestine/multivisceral, and some pancreas transplants. Bone marrow and cornea transplants aren't limited to approved facilities. Transplant coverage includes necessary tests, labs, and exams before surgery. It also includes immunosuppressive drugs (under certain conditions), follow-up care for you, and procurement of organs and tissues. Medicare pays for the costs for a living donor for a kidney transplant.
Transportation (Routine)	Medicare generally doesn't cover transportation to get routine health care. For more information, see Ambulance Services.
Travel Outside of the United States (Health Care Coverage During Travel)	Medicare generally doesn't cover health care while you are traveling outside the United States. Puerto Rico, the U.S. Virgin Islands, Guam, American Samoa, and the Northern Mariana Islands are considered part of the United States. There are some exceptions. In some cases, Medicare may pay for services that you get while on board a ship within the territorial waters adjoining the land areas of the United States. In rare cases, Medicare can pay for inpatient hospital services that you get in a foreign country. Medicare can pay only under the following circumstances: 1. You are in the United States when a medical emergency occurs and the foreign hospital is closer than the nearest United States hospital that can treat the emergency. 2. You are traveling through Canada without unreasonable delay by the most direct route between Alaska and another state when a medical emergency occurs and the Canadian hospital is closer than the nearest United States hospital that can treat the emergency. 3. You live in the United States and the foreign hospital is closer to your home than the nearest United States hospital that can treat your medical condition, regardless of whether an emergency exists. Medicare also pays for doctor and ambulance services you get in a foreign country as part of a covered inpatient hospital stay.
Walker/Wheelchair	Medicare covers power-operated vehicles (scooters), walkers, and wheelchairs as durable medical equipment that your doctor prescribes for use in your home. For more information, see Durable Medical Equipment. Power Wheelchair: You must have a face-to-face examination and a written prescription from a doctor or other treating provider before Medicare helps pay for a power wheelchair.
X-rays	Medicare covers medically necessary diagnostic X-rays that are ordered by your treating doctor. For more information, see Diagnostic Tests.

Source: U.S. Department of Health & Human Services Centers for Medicare & Medicaid Services (2007). Your Medicare benefits. Retrieved September 2, 2007 from http://www.medicare.gov/Publications/Pubs/pdf/10116.pdf

- The Medicare traditional plan previously described has undergone much scrutiny since its inception in 1965. From a government perspective, providing Medicare coverage to an increasingly larger cohort of older adults is challenging and has resulted in limited reimbursement. Attempts to resolve some of these issues, numerous changes, and additions to the traditional Medicare plan have evolved.
- Medigap is private (nongovernmental) health insurance available to Medicare recipients for purchase to help pay for what Medicare does not cover.
- Some of the health care expenses covered by Medigap include Medicare deductibles, co-pays (the additional amount of money that the patient must pay the health care provider), health care outside the United States, and medications.
- The federal government has set regulations that must be followed by the providers of these plans.
- There are 10 standard plans that must cover some of the essentials such as deductibles. However, each Medigap plan may also have additional benefits and set its own premiums.
- Many traditional Medicare recipients purchase a Medigap policy. However, some older Medicare patients cannot afford the monthly premiums for these supplemental plans.
- The Medicare Prescription Drug Improvement and Modernization Act of 2003 approved prescription discount drug cards for Medicare recipients. These cards are available to over 7 million of Medicare's 41 million participants. To be eligible for the discount cards, older adults must apply, and, depending on their income, a fee of $30 may be charged. The cards provide discounts on some, but not all, medications.
- Culture impacts health care reimbursement in that many older adults who have immigrated to the United States live their later lives with their adult children. Those who have not paid into the U.S. Social Security system must either buy into the Medicare system (the traditional health reimbursement program for older adults) or become eligible for Medicaid. However, legislation passed in the 1990s made it more difficult for older adults who were not U.S. citizens to access Medicaid, with the result that older adults may not have any way to pay for health care.

Medicare Managed Care, Prospective Payment Systems, and Other Medicare Systems

- Medicare Managed Care began a strong movement in the early 1990s in an attempt to lower the administrative costs associated with Medicare.
- Medicare recipients were asked to select a health maintenance organization (HMO) in which to receive their health care.
- Health care received through these HMOs would be paid for by Medicare.
- Unfortunately for the HMOs, older adults used considerably more health care services than Medicare reimbursed the HMO.

- Consequently, HMOs lost money, and, by 2000, many had withdrawn from the Medicare Managed Care business. While some HMOs still serve older adults in many parts of the country, many HMOs no longer take older adult Medicare clients.
- Because of the increasing cost of health care in the 1970s and 1980s, federal legislation in 1983 implemented a prospective payment system (PPS) that involved a set payment amount before care based on the diagnosis of the patient.
- This prospective payment system was based on defined diagnostic related groups (Sultz & Young, 1999). This system set a limit on the amount of money the hospital would be reimbursed for hospital stays.
- As a result of the implementation of the PPS system, older adults tend to receive more surgery and other treatments on an outpatient basis.
- While there are certainly positive aspects of this change in health care delivery—such as the ability to meet health care goals more effectively at home and the ability to remain free from the risks of hospitalization—should a problem arise, the need to transport to a facility with appropriate resources may be necessary, and the delay in accessing these services could increase both morbidity and mortality.
- In further attempts to repair the problems in the Medicare system, three newer alternatives have evolved:

  - Preferred provider organizations provide discounts to older adults who choose primary care providers and specialists who have agreed to accept Medicare assignment for patients.
  - Medicare fee-for-service plans contract with private providers to allow older adults to go to any Medicare-approved doctor or hospital that is willing to take them. Benefits of these plans are improved coverage, such as extra hospital days. However, providers must work with private insurance plans directly to determine coverage for the health care expenditures. Moreover, an additional premium may be involved.
  - Specialty plans to meet the diverse and comprehensive needs of older adults are currently being developed. More information on these plans will be available as they become more widely utilized among older adults.

Medicaid

- Medicaid, a combined federal and state payment system, varies from state to state, but it funds health care, including nursing home care, for low-income older adults.
- Medicaid is a governmental program aimed at improving access to health care for indigent individuals.
- Medicaid is a state-administered welfare program of health care for all ages. In fact, half of Medicaid recipients are children.
- To be eligible for Medicaid, older adults must meet specific income and asset guidelines put forth by their state.

- Older people who have minimal financial resources and who qualify for income assistance through a federal program called Supplemental Security Income (SSI) also become eligible for Medicaid health care benefits.
- Persons aged 65 and older may have Medicare benefits and also qualify for Medicaid.
- For older adults with limited assets and income, Medicaid may supplement Medicare benefits and pay for health care expenses not covered by Medicare, including medications, additional hospital or nursing home days, and durable medical equipment.
- For older adults who have both Medicare and Medicaid coverage for health care, Medicare is the primary payment system and Medicaid is secondary.
- The Centers for Medicare & Medicaid Services (2005) reports that Medicaid is currently the largest source of funding for health-related services for the poor in the United States.
- Medicaid was enacted by the same legislation as Medicare in 1965, also known as Title XIX of the Social Security Act.
- There is wide variability in covered medical expenses throughout the country.
- Each state establishes eligibility guidelines, allowable expenses, how much will be paid for these expenses, and how the program will be run within the state. Thus, there are as many different Medicaid programs as there are states. Mandated covered expenses for older adults include

  - Inpatient and outpatient hospital services
  - Physician services
  - Nursing home services
  - Home care services that are delivered to prevent nursing home stays
  - Laboratory and X-ray services

- Many state Medicaid programs provide extended coverage for home and community-based services if these services are keeping the older adult out of a covered nursing home stay that fall within a newer Medicaid program known as All-inclusive Care for the Elderly.
- The Personal Responsibility and Work Opportunity Reconciliation Act of 1996 welfare reform bill made legal resident aliens and other qualified aliens who entered the United States on or after that period ineligible for Medicaid for 5 years.
- If an older adult is a Medicaid recipient, payment for health care expenses is provided directly to the health care provider.
- Although Medicaid is used by all population groups in each state, the highest expenditures are made on behalf of older adults. While children average approximately $1,200 a year in Medicaid expenditure, older adults, who make up 9% of Medicaid recipients, average approximately $11,000 per person in annual Medicaid expenditures.

- Medicaid payments for long-term care services utilized primarily by older adults were approximately $37.2 billion in 2001 (Centers for Medicare & Medicaid Services, 2005).
- Medicaid has more enhanced coverage and fewer limitations than Medicare.

Long-Term Care Insurance

- Long-term care insurance is a relatively new concept designed to meet the needs of the growing elderly population.
- The likelihood of older adults requiring long-term care at some point in time in their lives is approximately 50% (Alexander, 2005).
- With an average stay of 19 months and an average cost of $30,000 per year, most older adults cannot afford to pay out of pocket for nursing home stays.
- Consequently, an illness that results in a nursing home stay has the potential to bankrupt most middle-income older adults.
- Long-term care insurance was developed by private insurance companies to meet the long-term and chronic health care needs of older adults.
- Long-term care insurance was designed to pay for long-term health services when multiple chronic health problems occur that require custodial care not covered by Medicare or other insurance.
- There are many advantages to owning a long-term care insurance policy. But, while insurance companies that offer long-term care policies are usually very ethical, they are essentially businesses with an interest in profit.
- Monthly premiums vary depending on one's age at the time of policy purchase, the length of coverage desired, the waiting period, and the desired amount of daily payments for health care expenses. Premiums are usually not fixed and may increase throughout the coverage period.
- In some cases, the premium may rise so high that older adults are no longer able to afford to pay. This may result in policy cancellation and loss of all previous monthly premiums, just when the policy benefits are needed to cover long-term nursing home, assisted living, or home care services.
- Long-term care insurance generally provides coverage for approved care in nursing facilities and assisted living.
- Care in the home by health care providers and community-based services such as care at adult day care centers are usually covered. Because the policies vary greatly, some services in these facilities may not be covered by long-term care policies.
- Long-term care insurance may be appropriate for middle-income individuals and couples who have too many financial assets to qualify for Medicaid but not enough assets to pay for long-term care.
- Because it has not been available until recently, most of the current cohort of the older adult population would be charged high premiums for

coverage. Thus, long-term care insurance is rarely used for paying for long-term health care among today's older adults.

- As baby boomers begin to consider their retirement years and plan for the future, the ability to purchase long-term care insurance and utilize it for payment of future health care expenses will increase.

Veteran's Benefits

- The Department of Veterans Affairs (VA) is a government entity that provides health care for veterans (military personnel who fought during a war).
- VA health care is provided through a network of VA medical centers, hospitals, and health facilities located across the country.
- Once eligibility has been determined, qualified veterans may receive health care for low or no cost.
- Eligibility for VA health care coverage, or the amount of coverage the veteran is entitled to, depends on several factors.
- Most active-duty military personnel who served in the Army, Navy, Air Force, Marines, or Coast Guard and were honorably discharged are eligible for VA health care coverage.
- Military reservists and National Guard members who served on active duty on order from the federal government may also be eligible for some VA health services.
- Eligibility for health care coverage is not limited to those who served in combat.
- The Veterans' Health Care Eligibility Reform Act of 1996 was developed to clarify eligibility for VA health care coverage and improve health benefits for qualified beneficiaries.
- The legislation resulted in the development of the current Uniform Benefits Package—a standard health benefits plan generally available to all veterans.
- Once eligibility has been approved, VA health coverage under the Uniform Benefits Package is comprehensive and provides for both inpatient and outpatient coverage at VA medical centers and facilities nationwide and abroad.
- Outpatient clinics provide physician services, primary and preventive care, diagnostic testing (including laboratory tests), minor surgery, and other needed benefits such as prescription medications.
- The VA will also pay for hearing aids and other services after a small deductible has been met. This service is available even if the prescriptions were written by a physician other than at the VA hospital or facility.
- Veterans with service-connected health problems are usually given priority status, but, because all veterans may receive health care at these clinics, waiting times for appointments and services may be long.

References

Alexander, R. (Ed). (2005). *Avoiding fraud when buying long-term care insurance: A guide for consumers and their families.* Retrieved May 14, 2005, from http://consumerlawpage.com/article/insure.shtml#intro

Centers for Medicare and Medicaid Services. (2005). *Medicaid: A brief overview.* Retrieved May 12, 2005, from http://www.cms.hhs.gov/publications/overview-medicare-medicaid/default4.asp

Sultz, H. A., & Young, K. M. (1999). *Health care USA* (2nd ed.). Gaithersburg, MD: Aspen.

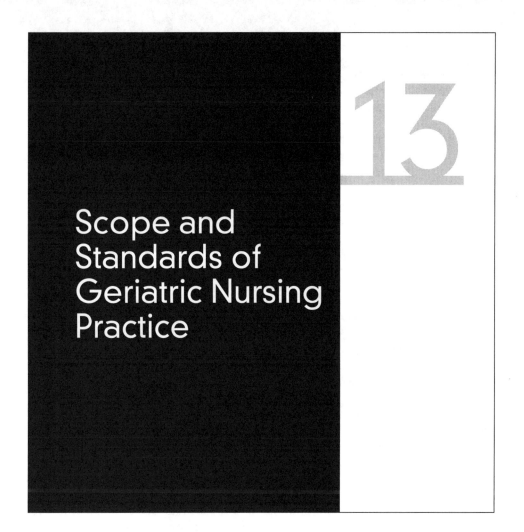

13

Scope and Standards of Geriatric Nursing Practice

Leadership and Management

All gerontological nurses must be leaders in making sure they provide the highest quality care to the older adults they are responsible for, be it direct bedside care or facilitating patient care by others. Nurses need to be able to take on the following roles: creative thinker, risk taker, patient advocate, empowering others to lead, change maker, visionary, excellent communicator, and steward (Grossman & Valiga, 2005). It is imperative that nurses be committed to making a difference, facilitating followers in gaining leadership ability, and realizing that every nurse must lead in the chaotic and challenging U.S. health care system. It is significant to understand the differences in leadership types such as transformational and transactional leadership. Transactional leadership tends to be evident in health care, because it involves getting the job accomplished and is very task focused. Transformational leadership involves more of an inspirational sharing between leaders and followers where both groups are motivated and energized to perform beyond their job descriptions. Sashkin and Sashkin (2003) identify the following skills that characterize transformational leadership:

- Ability to identify co-workers' feelings
- Ability to motivate others
- Ability to manage one's emotions with co-workers

By having a transformational leadership style, nurses can make a difference in their practice. Bennis (2007) suggests that exemplary leaders have six competencies that are commonly evident. They

- Create sense of mission
- Motivate followers to work with them on the mission
- Develop a social ambience for their followers
- Create trust and optimism
- Develop others to lead
- Obtain results

Nurses working with older adults need to practice good management, which is described as being able to manage the staff and the budget, follow the organization's policies and procedures, and generate high-quality care. They are responsible for assessing, analyzing, planning, implementing, and evaluating all of the services that are part of their unit's or, in some cases, their agencies' health care delivery.

Managers need to be effective decision makers, reflective critical thinkers, excellent time managers, and fiscal agents. Using cost-benefit analysis, nurse managers can assess the financial resources projected for costs and benefits of new programs or equipment for their unit(s). They also need to be able to foster professional development in their staff, manage conflict in all areas of their unit as well as regarding intra-agency unit problems. They are responsible for building teams of professional and unlicensed assistant personnel in order to have cost-efficient and effective health care delivery on their unit.

Nurse managers need to be able to manage conflict by assisting people with their communication style. They need to encourage active listening and make sure that the team understands and shares the goal of providing the highest quality patient care. Such skills include

- Being able to identify how individuals manage conflict
- Having self-awareness of how one manages conflict
- Engaging in active listening
- Mutual resolution so that win-win is the overall outcome

It is essential to incorporate all of the staff when making decisions so that there will be more buy-in, and the new idea will be successful when it is implemented. The same goes for any changes that need to be made. An example of good strategizing in planning a change is explained in Sherwood's (2006) article on experiential learning, where everyone on the unit had the opportunity to participate in making the change and having a say in what was going to happen on the unit. Due to the involvement of everyone on the staff, this change was successfully accepted.

Quality Improvement

Few quality improvement programs operate on a consistent basis in long-term care facilities; this is thought to be impacted by staff turnover and limited training among many nurse administrators in these institutions (Adams-Wendling & Lee, 2005). Quality improvement programs must be established at long-term care facilities so that outcome data can be measured and so it can be determined whether the facility is providing a high-quality standard of care. It is imperative that measurable outcome data are collected and tracked on clinical indicators such as falls, medication errors, skin ulcers, infection rates, and admission/transfer rates to and from nursing homes to hospitals so that patients can be assured that they are receiving the highest possible quality care.

Accreditation by the Joint Commission (previously known as the Joint Commission of Hospital Accrediting Organization) involves various audits that are assessed to validate the data that patients are experiencing high-quality care. Facilities are also assessed for performance and continued improvement in care. Audits to assess outcome, process, and structure must be done on a routine basis so that the facilities can be accredited successfully. The Centers for Medicare & Medicaid Services have similar conditions of participation that agencies caring for patients must demonstrate.

Staff nurses must be aware of the hospital quality assurance indicators and be able to identify patients who are at high risk so more careful scrutiny can be assigned. If certain problems regarding medication or falls are occurring frequently, then interventions need to be implemented to prevent recurrences. In-services should be planned that focus on high-frequency, high-risk, and problem areas to identify the areas that staff feel they need to learn more about in order to promote high quality and safe care in the hospital, unit, or facility. It is always prudent to conduct a needs assessment in order to determine the learning needs of staff so that they can be successful with their job duties. It is significant for nurses to be aware of the multiple assessment tools that are available to assist in the process of evaluating care and patient outcomes: the Older Americans Resources and Services Assessment measures economic resources, mental health, and activities of daily living; and the Functional Status Assessment measures a person's ability to perform his or her functions such as activities of daily living.

Due to the increased focus on the Institute of Medicine's (2001) findings regarding patient safety in hospitals, today it is even more imperative to have frequent quality improvement checks of patient care standards, and this pertains to long term facilities, too. *Crossing the Quality Chasm: A New Health System for the 21st Century* (Institute of Medicine, 2001) provides several guidelines to assist institutions with changes that will improve the safety culture. For example, several of these guidelines describe precepts for patient-centered care:

- Care is customized according to the patient's needs and values.
- The patient is the source of control.
- Knowledge is shared, and information flows freely.
- Transparency is necessary.
- Needs are anticipated.

Kohn, Corrigan, and Donaldson (2000) also describe the significance of providing patient-centered care. Certainly, the Joint Commission's (2008a, 2008b) National Patient Safety Goals are important to review and implement with the care of older adults. Johnstone and Kanitsaki (2006) cite statistics supporting errors in health care. They report that approximately 4% to 16% of patients experience harm as a result of human error in hospitals and that 50% of these errors could have been prevented.

There are many ideas that can be adapted from industries other than health care that can assist in improving care. For example, Six Sigma, a quality improvement method that uses data analysis and standardized formulas to eliminate problems has increased productivity and success at several corporations and would be easily adaptable to health care settings. Its philosophy is to prevent mistakes, waste, and redoing work.

Organizational Concepts

Nurses working with older adults in long-term care facilities can attend professional development classes on a variety of topics, such as the organizational structure, philosophy, goals, and objectives of the agency. Generally, the nurse manager of a unit in a long-term care facility is the director of nursing within the organizational structure and is responsible for all members of the unit staff. The facility's organizational structure illustrates the lines of communication and authority from the top administrator to the unlicensed assistive personnel and environmental assistants (Huber, 2006).

An agency's mission is the purpose and reason for its existence. The philosophy incorporates the values that guide the actions of the organization. The strategic plan identifies the long-range planning for the next 3 to 5 years. The goals and objectives of the agency describe the actions that will be taken to accomplish the strategic plan. There may be individualized unit goals that stem from the overall agency goals. The policies and procedures of an organization describe the exact processes of action that nurses should take for implementing all policies and procedures at the institution.

Professional Development

Katz et al. (2004) describe the professional nurse as having multiple roles such as provider, health educator, advocate, case manager, change agent, manager, leader, and several similar roles at the advanced level of practice. They further define the profession as being focused on delivering holistic care to individuals, families, and communities for actual and potential health problems. All nurses have a responsibility to attend continuing education programs and maintain their competency in practice. Many nurses have peer mentors and preceptors to assist them in maintaining their professional expertise and role models or mentors to assist them in accomplishing their career goals.

The nursing profession was the first of the health care disciplines to develop gerontological care standards for their members to demonstrate and be tested for their level of expertise. The Gerontological Nurse certification (for which you are likely preparing) offered by the American Nurses Credentialing Center (2007) is an example of how nursing standards of care have been developed.

Nurses can access best practices protocols in gerontology through journals, professional organizations, gerontology conferences, and Web sites such as the John A. Hartford Foundation Institute for Geriatric Nursing (http://www.hartfordign.org).

Legal and Ethical Issues

Regulatory Guidelines

Patients receiving care in any institution are cared for under the auspice of the Patients' Bill of Rights. Many agencies have patient ombudsmen who advocate for patients' rights. Many states have enacted right-to-die laws, and patients are able to declare their desires regarding end-of-life care in advanced directives. There are statutes that control access to patient records and guarantee patient privacy, such as the Health Insurance Portability and Accountability Act.

In many instances, nurses must delegate care to others in order to accomplish the care management for older adults in long-term care and assisted living facilities. Knowing how and what can be delegated must be carefully assessed by the registered nurse. The National Council of State Boards of Nursing (NCSBN, 2005) developed the following framework of the Five Rights of Delegation that can be helpful to nurses when determining who can perform what duties:

- Right task
- Right circumstances
- Right person
- Right direction/communication
- Right supervision

The NCSBN also delineates a process for applying the five rights of delegation when assessing a nurse's role determined by the Nurse Practice Act. Any care that a registered nurse (RN) delegates to a nursing assistant or licensed practical nurse (LPN) that is not part of the job description needs to be supervised by the RN. If the task delegated is one for which the LPN or nurse assistant has been trained, is one in which he or she can demonstrate competence, and it is in the scope of his or her practice, then the LPN or nurse assistant is accountable for his or her actions.

Ethical Principles and Decision Making

Nurses must follow ethical principles as they practice and make decisions regarding patient care. For example, every nurse should follow these principles:

- Beneficence—Nurses should always do good and prevent harm to all patients.

- Nonmalfeasance—Nurses must state their duty not to inflict harm.
- Veracity—Nurses must always uphold the truth.
- Utilitarianism—Nurses must make the decision that is positive for the most people involved.

Nurses must use the Code of Ethics for Nurses when they practice. This framework describes the ethical and professional values of a nurse as developed by the American Nurses Association (2001). It is important that nurses practice so that patients can be autonomous and maintain the right to make their own choices. Nurses must uphold the values that society regards as desirable (Cherry & Jacob, 2008).

Research

The research process is becoming very evident in all practice areas. Nurses are expected to be aware of the general aspects of conducting research. In fact, nurses must be able to interpret research in the literature so they can use the findings in their practice. It is important for nurses to have a general competence in understanding the quality of a research study. All nurses must understand that research is a systematic inquiry that follows disciplined methods to answer problems (Polit & Beck, 2008). Such an inquiry would include the following concepts:

Problem being researched—What is the background of the problem being researched?

Literature review—Has the author reviewed the appropriate data? Does the literature review span the findings published over the last 5 years?

Purpose of the research—Does the article have a specific purpose for conducting the research? Are there research questions identified that relate to the overall purpose?

Informed consent—Have the researchers fully informed the participants of the study about what they are going to be asked to do? For example, have non-English speaking participants been communicated with in a language they understand regarding the research study? Have the authors obtained Institutional Review Board (IRB) permission to conduct the study? Often the researchers are from universities, and they will apply for IRB consent from their university. Other times, the agency (such as a visiting nurse agency or a long-term care facility) have their own IRB from which the researchers will need to obtain approval before beginning the study.

Sample—Is the sample large enough? Does the sample represent the various types of people among the general population that are relevant in studying this problem? If the sample of study participants represents the general population, then the findings of the research are considered generalizable to the population.

Data collection—Is the study sample randomly selected or is it biased by the researchers' data collection methods? Is it a convenience sample (that is, were the survey participants chosen from one specific nursing home rather than a random selection of people from multiple nursing homes)?

Tool—Was the research tool standardized and reliable (that is, does the tool measure what it supposed to measure), and does the tool have validity (the findings are unbiased and well grounded)? Has this tool been shown to have consistent reliability and validity?

Results—Are the results relevant to clinical practice? Are they going to make a difference in practice?

Data analysis—Are the findings statistically significant at the .05 level or .01 level? Or are they not statistically significant?

Discussion of findings and implications for clinical practice—Has the purpose of the study been accomplished? What else needs to be done?

Evidence-Based Practice

All nursing practice is expected to be based on emerging evidence from research, which is called evidence-based practice. Polit and Beck (2008) describe evidence-based practice as using the best possible clinical evidence to make clinical decisions for patient care. Evidence-based practice has determined that some of the "tried and true" nursing methods that have been learned from either nursing school or practice are not the best way of practicing. The best practices for gerontology can be accessed at multiple Web sites, such as the John A. Hartford Foundation Institute for Geriatric Nursing, http://www.hartfordign.org.

References

Adams-Wendling, L., & Lee, L. (2005). Quality improvement in nursing facilities: A nursing leadership perspective. *Journal of Gerontological Nursing, 31*(11), 36–41.

American Nurses Association. (2001). *Code of ethics for nurses with interpretive statements.* Washington, DC: American Nurses Publishing.

American Nurses Credential Center. (2007). Gerontological nurse certification. Retrieved September 22, 2007, from http://www.nursecredentialing.org

Bennis, W. (2007). The challenges of leadership in the modern world. *American Psychologist, 62*(1), 2–5.

Cherry, B., & Jacob, S. (2008). *Contemporary nursing: Issues, trends, and management* (4th ed.). St. Louis, MO: Elsevier.

Grossman, S., & Valiga, T. (2005). *The new leadership challenge: Creating the future of nursing* (2nd ed.). Philadelphia: F. A. Davis.

Huber, D. (2006). *Leadership and nursing care management* (3rd ed.). Philadelphia: Saunders.

Institute of Medicine. (2001). *Crossing the quality chasm: A new health system for the 21st century.* Washington, DC: National Academies Press.

Johnstone, M., & Kanitsaki, O. (2006). The moral imperative of designating patient safety and quality care as a national nursing research priority. *Collegian, 13*(1), 5–9.

Joint Commission. (2008a). *2008 National patient safety goals.* Retrieved March 26, 2008, from http://www.jointcommission.org/PatientSafety/NationalPatientSafetyGoals

Joint Commission. (2008b). *2008 National patient safety goals: Critical access hospital program.* Retrieved March 26, 2008, from http://www.jointcommission.org/PatientSafety/National PatientSafetyGoals/08_cah_npsgs.htm

Katz, J., Carter, C., Bishop, J., & Lyman Kravits, S. (2004). *Keys to nursing success* (2nd ed.). Columbus, OH: Pearson/Prentice Hall.

Kohn, L., Corrigan, J., & Donaldson, M. (2000). *To err is human: Building a safer health system.* Washington, DC: National Academies Press.

National Council of State Boards of Nursing. (2005). Working with others: A position paper. Retrieved September 8, 2007, from http://www.ncsbn.org

Polit, D., & Beck, C. (2008). *Nursing research: Generating and assessing evidence for nursing practice* (8th ed.). Philadelphia: Lippincott Williams & Wilkins.

Sashkin, M., & Sashkin, M. (2003). *Leadership that matters: The critical factors for making a difference in people's lives and organizations' success.* San Francisco: Berrett and Koehler.

Sherwood, G. (2006). Management and leadership in nursing and health care: An experiential approach. *Journal of Continuing Education in Nursing, 37*(4), 191.

POSTTEST

1. You are performing an eye assessment of an 80-year-old client. Which of the following findings is considered abnormal?

   a. Loss of outer hair on the eyebrows due to a decrease in hair follicles.
   b. The presence of arcus senilus seen around the cornea.
   c. A decrease in tear production.
   d. Unequal pupillary constriction in response to light.

2. When discussing the increase in the number of older adults in the United States, use the term:

   a. Graying of America
   b. Maximum life span
   c. Life expectancy
   d. Total time until death

3. Tertiary prevention activities are designed to:

   a. Prevent disease before it occurs.
   b. Detect disease at an earlier, more treatable stage.
   c. Manage disease, so it does not get worse.
   d. Eradicate all disease from the nation.

4. An 85-year-old man complains of nausea, sweating, and feeling "very weak" over the last 8 hours. He presents in the emergency department with a history of gastroesophageal reflux disease, coronary artery disease, and coronary artery bypass graft within the last 3 months. He has no other complaints. After taking vital signs, which are stable, your first action would be to:

   a. Take a finger stick to assess blood sugar.
   b. Perform an electrocardiogram.
   c. Draw blood for chemistry profile, CBC with differential.
   d. Contact the geriatrician on call.

5. A 68-year-old woman was seen by her cardiologist for palpitations. She was put on a beta blocker and told to return for follow-up 1 week after taking a stress test. The beta blocker's action:

   a. Increases consistency of heart rate
   b. Increases contractility and decreases heart rate

    c. Decreases chance of dysrhythmia

    d. Decreases contractility and increases heart rate

6. Mary Palmer has been admitted to your unit with congestive heart failure. Which of the following symptoms are most likely to be present in this 93-year-old?

    a. Cough

    b. Decreased cognitive status

    c. Fever

    d. Sudden onset pedal edema

7. Herzberg is an example of what type of theory?

    a. Nursing grand theory

    b. Sociological aging theory

    c. Motivational theory

    d. Eccentricity theory

8. Mr. Gladbottle is complaining of pain, for which he needs medication. All of the following normal changes of aging should be considered when administering the medication, *except:*

    a. Decreased hydrogen/oxygen breakdown

    b. Decreased absorption from gastrointestinal track

    c. Decreased metabolism of medications

    d. Decreased renal clearance

9. Older men are at high risk for stomach cancer. In order to have early detection they should be taught to recognize the symptoms, which include:

    a. Abdominal distention, lower abdominal cramping, and blood in stool

    b. Epigastric discomfort, increased flatus, and mid-abdominal cramping

    c. Anorexia, nausea, and epigastric discomfort

    d. Dysphagia, excessive belching, and increased flatus

10. You have just admitted an 88-year-old man to the long-term care facility. He is on several medications, including allopurinol (Zyloprim) and bethanechol (Urecholine), which are for:

    a. Arthritis

    b. Amyotrophic lateral sclerosis

    c. Gout

    d. Polyarteritis

11. A new staff nurse is orienting to the long-term care facility. The staff development coordinator will be sure to include time for the new nurse to review the institution's:

    a. Plan for developing new funding for the facility

    b. Listing of each staff member's salary

    c. Mission, philosophy, and goals of the organization

    d. The next 6 months' scheduling of nursing assistants on each unit

12. A 68-year-old and resident of an assisted living facility complains of muscle aches and loss of range of motion in multiple joints, especially in his left knee. He says he is sexually active and has multiple partners. His temperature is 99.1°; he has no tophi on his left knee, but it is warm and swollen. The etiology of his knee pain is:

a. Severe osteopenia or osteoporosis
b. Septic arthritis secondary to gonorrhea and chlamydia
c. Sarcoidosis
d. Osteomyelitis

13. The *absence* of which of the following symptoms makes diagnosis of pneumonia difficult in older adults?

a. Bradycardia
b. Tachycardia
c. Cough
d. Cyanosis

14. The nurse manager of a geriatric unit has been having trouble motivating the staff on her unit and recently received low patient and nurse satisfaction scores. The other RNs on this unit are transferring to other units whenever there are open positions. This manager is noted for her authoritarian leadership and strong task-oriented style. She reflects the following type of leadership:

a. Democratic
b. Transformational
c. Transactional
d. Laissez-faire

15. It may take several weeks for the postherpetic pain secondary to herpes zoster experienced by many older adults to subside. Therefore, it is recommended that a pain medication and the following therapy be used:

a. Magnet therapy
b. Continued acyclovir (Zovirax)
c. Meperidine (Demerol)
d. Capsaicin cream

16. A 77-year-old man presents to the emergency department in acute pain. He says he has new onset left leg pain and that his leg is really swollen with erythematous streaks. He is diagnosed with:

a. Gout
b. Rheumatoid arthritis
c. Cellulitis
d. Fibromyalgia

17. If a study is said to use a random sampling, this means the sample was:

a. Representative of the average American
b. Chosen on the basis of convenience

c. Determined using clustering technique to ensure homogeneity
d. Selected so that each member of a population has an equal probability of being included

18. A 77-year-old woman is admitted for shortness of breath, muscular aches, fever, and severe dehydration. She has been away visiting her daughter and missed her regular annual exam. Most likely, she did not have:

a. Influenza vaccine
b. Pneumovax vaccine
c. Pulmonary profile
d. Electrolyte and renal function screen

19. The degree to which a patient follows a treatment regimen could best be defined as:

a. Compliance
b. Adherence
c. Deliverance
d. Holism

20. A 79-year-old man has been taking proton pump inhibitors for over 5 years for his gastritis. He recently complained of numbness in his hands and feet, fatigue, confusion, and soreness in his mouth and gums. You ask the nurse practitioner to order the following to determine the etiology of his complaints:

a. B_{12} level
b. Toxicity screen
c. Sedimentation rate
d. Cortisol

21. Due to the fact that there can be under- and overestimates of an individual's abilities, it is best to use the following for the primary source of information in an older adult assessment:

a. Primary care provider
b. The spouse or child of the older adult
c. The older adult
d. The executive of the older adult's estate

22. Restraints should rarely be used in long-term care facilities. However, which of the following situations is an acceptable reason for using restraints on an older adult?

a. When the patient wants to get out of bed and go to the bathroom several times a night
b. When the patient is restless and has no order for a sedative
c. When the patient becomes agitated after meals
d. To ensure the physical safety of the patient or other patients

23. Posttransplant, the chance for developing acute graft-versus-host disease tends to fall between:

a. The first 20 days posttransplant
b. Within the first 24 hours posttransplant

c. Between 30 and 50 days posttransplant
d. Within the first week posttransplant

24. Which of the following points would the nurse include in teaching an older adult beginning an exercise program?

a. Begin an exercise program with 30 to 60 minutes of vigorous exercise each day.
b. Avoid drinking water when exercising.
c. Keep a daily written log of exercise and include type of exercise, time of exercise, and the intensity of exercise.
d. Dizziness is common when exercising and should be ignored.

25. To obtain a patient's informed consent to participate in a research study, the researcher must obtain approval from:

a. Nurses working with the patient
b. Patient's family members
c. Long-term care facility attorney
d. Institutional Review Board

26. An 88-year-old man complains of burning on the soles of his feet. He has a complete physical examination and has no other significant findings. His laboratory work returns with a decrease in:

a. Vitamin C
b. Vitamin B_{12}
c. Iron
d. Potassium

27. Mrs. Crotwell is a 90-year-old woman who has been hospitalized with a medical diagnosis of osteoporosis. Which of the following is most likely her primary form of insurance?

a. COBRA
b. Medicare
c. Medicaid
d. HUSKY

28. A 77-year-old patient has just been admitted to the coronary care unit for a myocardial infarction. His blood sugar is 165, but he has no history of diabetes mellitus. The treatment to manage his elevated blood sugar will consist of:

a. NPH (neutral protamine Hagedorn) and regular insulin with a sliding scale
b. Lente and regular insulin with a sliding scale
c. Subcutaneous regular insulin with a sliding scale
d. Basal and bolus insulin

29. The end of life is often associated with which of the following psychological symptoms among older adults?

a. Anxiety
b. Cough

c. Shortness of breath

d. Pain

30. An 81-year-old man has been experiencing some memory loss over the last year, but today he got lost driving to his son's home. He has had various laboratory tests, neuroimaging, and cognitive testing and has been diagnosed with Alzheimer's disease. Due to his increasing dementia, he is being discharged to his son's home. The priority intervention that must be promoted is:

a. Protection from injury

b. Behavior modification

c. Independence with activities of daily living

d. Memory restoration

31. The purpose of the Health Insurance Portability and Accountability Act (HIPAA) is to:

a. Provide reimbursement for prescriptions.

b. Set up insurance policies for emergencies.

c. Provide older adults guaranteed access to health care.

d. Guarantee patient privacy.

32. In the continuity theory of aging:

a. Successful aging is dependent on the individual's developmental patterns throughout life.

b. Aging should be denied as long as possible.

c. Cells divide continually a predetermined number of times, and then death occurs.

d. Products of oxidation result in a breakdown of cell, and the body slowly begins to age.

33. Many older adults have painful hips and knees and have osteoarthritis. An appropriate intervention for them is:

a. Application of heat and/or cold—whichever is effective

b. NSAIDS with food every 2 hours

c. Steroids BID

d. Cortisone injections BID

34. Older adults with pneumonia are 3 to 5 times more likely than younger patients with pneumonia to experience the following

a. Cardiovascular collapse

b. Complications leading to death

c. Fever > 105°F

d. Acute renal failure

35. A characteristic of delirium is:

a. Intellectual dysfunction that occurs slowly and lasts for longer than 6 months

b. Decreased severity at nighttime

   c. Disorientation

   d. A progressive decline in memory

36. A 66-year-old presents with a purple-colored papular rash on his face. He is HIV positive and states that the rash is worsening, he has never experienced it before, and, although painless, it is causing concern. The rash is:

   a. Psoriasis

   b. Tinea capitus

   c. Impetigo

   d. Kaposi's sarcoma

37. A 77-year-old man has recently been diagnosed with beginning heart failure. He will most likely be prescribed the following:

   a. Digoxin

   b. ACE inhibitor

   c. Calcium channel blocker

   d. Beta blocker

38. A 75-year-old man is sightseeing in Arizona and finds that he is extremely thirsty in the hot climate. This is due to less ability to conserve fluid and concentrate urine. Therefore, one would expect:

   a. Increased glomerular filtration rate

   b. Decreased blood urea nitrogen and creatinine

   c. Decreased glomerular filtration rate

   d. Increased erythropoiten

39. Primary prevention activities are designed to:

   a. Prevent disease before it occurs.

   b. Detect disease at an earlier, more treatable stage.

   c. Manage disease, so it does not get worse.

   d. Eradicate all disease from the nation.

40. Common musculoskeletal problems for older adults include:

   a. Paget's disease and osteomyelitis

   b. Bunions and corns on feet

   c. Osteoarthritis and osteoporosis

   d. Rheumatoid arthritis and plantar fasciitis

41. Older adults often don't report pain because

   a. They believe that pain is a normal part of aging.

   b. They are afraid of what the pain might mean.

   c. They don't want to bother the nurse.

   d. All of the above.

42. Older adults tend to have increased dental problems due to:

   a. Periodontal disease

   b. Changes in pH of saliva

    c. Decreased fluid needs

    d. Less mucus excreted from salivary glands

43. Ways in which geriatric nurses may help older patients to fulfill their spiritual needs at the end of life may include:

    a. Ignore spiritual needs because these are best managed by other team members.

    b. Focus on pain management.

    c. Focus on maintaining adequate oxygenation.

    d. Encourage religious and spiritual practices at the end of life.

44. Practice that focuses on making decisions clinically using the best evidence available is called:

    a. Applied research practice

    b. Research utilization practice

    c. Evidence-based practice

    d. Empirical evidence practice

45. A 66-year-old man has recently been diagnosed with Meniere's disease and is experiencing another episode. His symptoms will include:

    a. Decreased hearing and difficulty with balance

    b. Pain in the outer ear and itchiness

    c. Shrill sounds upon talking and decreased hearing

    d. Dizziness and tinnitus

46. Older adults suffering from early dementia due to Alzheimer's disease are generally prescribed a cholinesterase inhibitor. The action of these drugs is to:

    a. Decrease catecholamine surges

    b. Increase the brain's level of acetylcholine

    c. Decrease serotonin uptake

    d. Increase norepinephrine levels

47. The organizational structure of any facility represents the:

    a. Line of authority from the administrator to the unlicensed assistive personnel

    b. Line of authority for the nursing personnel only

    c. Process by which the organization is departmentalized

    d. Categories of employees

48. Title III of the Older Americans Act facilitated the start of:

    a. Centers for Medicare & Medicaid Services

    b. AARP

    c. Area Agencies on Aging

    d. Gerontological Society of America

49. 40% to 60% of older adults have anemia due to iron deficiency or some chronic illness. Additionally, many medications can cause anemia, such as

the following drug category, which can cause gastrointestinal bleeding if not taken with food:

a. Anticonvulsants
b. Antihypertensives
c. NSAIDs
d. Diuretics

50. The temperature response of older adults to infection:

a. Is about the same as that of a young child
b. Varies widely because of the loss of subcutaneous fat and muscle tissue
c. Is always lower than that of younger adults
d. Depends on the type of thermometer used

51. A 73-year-old woman has osteoarthritis in multiple joints. She has an especially difficult time with fine motor work and has recently been diagnosed with:

a. Veritas erythema
b. Bouthard nodules
c. Heberden's nodes
d. Hallus valgus

52. One of the most influential advocacy groups for older adults is:

a. Centers for Medicare & Medicaid Services
b. AARP
c. Association on Aging
d. Gerontological Society of America

53. Geriatric nursing interventions in environments of care that can be used to address nursing diagnosis:

a. Are nursing actions that will assist the patient to meet the identified goals
b. Must be broad enough so that any member of the health care team can modify them if necessary
c. Are based on the medical diagnosis
d. Organize the data obtained in the assessment

54. The guidelines used to determine appropriate and correct dosages for medications for older adults is:

a. Coggs Criteria
b. Glasgow Scale
c. Beers Criteria
d. Ramsey's Scale

55. Many variables cause the increased risk of incontinence in older adults. Which of the following is a physiological factor of aging that impacts one's ability to have urinary continence?

a. Decreased ability to mobilize
b. Decreased cognition

    c. Decreased bladder capacity

    d. Depression

56. Which of these statements, if made by the older adult, would be most likely to be an indicator of depression?

    a. "I feel like I have accomplished something today."

    b. "I am just too tired to do anything."

    c. "I would like to visit my daughter."

    d. "My life has had many ups and downs."

57. An 83-year-old man presents with hyperlipidemia with the following laboratory results: TC 242, HDL 54, LDL 168, and TG 110. He has well-controlled hypertension and no other history. Which of the parameters should be focused on for management?

    a. HDL should be higher.

    b. LDL should be less than 100.

    c. Triglycerides should be lower.

    d. Total cholesterol should be around 240.

58. The following would be an appropriate activity for the RN to delegate to the unlicensed assistive personnel:

    a. Medication administration

    b. Nutritional assessment

    c. Bathing

    d. Admission documentation

59. Secondary prevention activities are designed to:

    a. Prevent disease before it occurs.

    b. Detect disease at an earlier, more treatable stage.

    c. Manage disease, so it does not get worse.

    d. Eradicate all disease from the nation.

60. A set of national health objectives designed to guide the health promotion activities of the United States is known as:

    a. Healthy People 1998

    b. Healthy People 2010

    c. A Sick Nation

    d. Blueprint for Health

61. Stress incontinence is common among older adults who can benefit from doing specific exercises such as:

    a. Bicellular stretches

    b. Detrussor splints

    c. Kegel exercises

    d. Perineum exercises

62. Approximately 20% of older adults experience restless legs syndrome. The following has been identified to exacerbate the condition:

    a. Excessive caffeine intake

    b. Folate deficiency

    c. Osteoarthritis

    d. Hypertension

63. Durable power of attorney provides which information if a patient should experience a terminal condition or a permanent state of unconsciousness?

    a. Written information describing the patient's desires for life-sustaining treatment

    b. Names a person for making health care decisions on behalf of the patient

    c. Provides information for the distribution of the patient's financial assets

    d. Provides for terminal care at the end of life

64. Older adults tend to have increased pulse pressures due to their:

    a. Decreased diastolic blood pressure

    b. Increased cardiac output

    c. Increased blood flow

    d. Decreased systolic blood pressure

65. An 81-year-old man has been experiencing temporal headaches and has been seen by his physician and diagnosed with temporal arteritis. He has most likely been prescribed:

    a. Azithromycin (Z pak)

    b. Ibuprofen (Advil)

    c. Prednisone

    d. Sumatriptan (Imitrex)

66. A 67-year-old man presents with red blotches, papules, and pustules on his face, especially over his chin and cheek areas. He says he does not remember ever having this problem before. This is most likely:

    a. Folliculitis

    b. Acne vulgaris

    c. Eczema

    d. Rosacea

67. A 76-year-old woman is postop craniotomy due to a benign tumor. She is febrile, has odorous drainage, and her incision is erythematous and indurated. You suspect she is infected and find that your older patients often experience infection postoperatively. This is due to:

    a. Fewer killer T cells in the immunologic system

    b. Inflammation due to increased cytokines

    c. Weaker neutrophil response to infection

    d. Cortisol deficiency

68. Health care costs for older adults have increased greatly as a result of which of the following factors?

    a. Increased technology

    b. Decreased educational levels of the elderly

    c. Decreased numbers of older adults

    d. The nursing shortage

69. It is most important to teach older adults with type 2 diabetes about the relationship of postprandial glucose levels and:

    a. Carbohydrates

    b. Fats

    c. Proteins

    d. Iron

70. In discussing the biological theories of aging, the nurse would include information on which of the following theories?

    a. The "wear and tear" theory

    b. The disengagement theory

    c. The continuity theory

    d. The activity theory

71. Measurements for accreditation are performed to assess quality of care in all hospitals and patient care facilities. What are these measurements called?

    a. Geriatric benchmarks

    b. Outcome, process, and structure

    c. Criteria for health of older adults

    d. Geriatric care standards

72. It is not uncommon for older adults who experience influenza to have persistent problems afterward such as:

    a. Anemia, chest discomfort, and cough

    b. Lack of energy, fatigue, and malaise

    c. Fatigue, anemia, and myalgia

    d. Malaise, fever, and cough

73. It is essential to realize that older adults must get an adequate dietary intake of the following element due to the fact that aging causes a decrease in absorption of this element in the gastrointestinal system:

    a. Potassium

    b. Sodium

    c. Hydrogen

    d. Iron

74. Mr. and Mrs. Suhul live in an assisted living facility and rarely leave their apartment. They have recently said that they feel depressed and lethargic and ask you about the facility's social activities. You suggest that they:

    a. Make appointments with the psychiatrist.

    b. Sign up for an exercise class, get some sun, and do yoga.

    c. Add more protein to their diets.

    d. Get a vitamin C supplement.

75. An older patient is preparing for discharge on warfarin (Coumadin) 5 mg orally every day. He asks you if he should continue with his multivitamin when he gets home. Your response is:

    a. "It is fine to take a multivitamin daily."
    b. "If there is no vitamin K in it, you can take it."
    c. "You should take two multivitamins daily."
    d. "It is best to take the multivitamin before you go to sleep."

76. In assessing pain in older adults, nurses must realize that:

    a. Older adults are quicker to report pain than younger adults.
    b. Pain is a normal consequence of aging.
    c. An elderly person may not exhibit outward signs of pain even when he or she is actually experiencing pain.
    d. Pain is rated on a scale of 0 to 10, with 10 being no feelings of pain and 0 being the most severe pain.

77. Older adults are frequently diagnosed with anemia of chronic disease, which is commonly seen with the following:

    a. Cardiovascular and pulmonary disease
    b. Renal and neurological problems
    c. Malignancies and tuberculosis
    d. Musculoskeletal and neurological problems

78. Nurses must complete a core set of screening and assessment elements that form the foundation of the comprehensive assessment for their home care residents. This assessment tool is called the:

    a. Minimum Data Set
    b. OASIS Assessment
    c. Resident Assessment Set
    d. Maximum Dependency Scale

79. Some older adults withhold medical information or details about their living arrangements, because they:

    a. May feel the care provider is not really interested in all of the details
    b. May not realize that some of this information would be helpful for planning their care
    c. May not remember all of the details of their medical history or living arrangements
    d. All of the above

80. Some older adults manifest changes in their skin that appear as light brown macules on the dorsum of their hand, wrist, and forearm called:

    a. Actinic keratosis
    b. Skin tags
    c. Rosacea
    d. Seborrheic dermatitis

81. Mr. H., an 81-year-old man, has an HDL of 75. Your teaching for him would include instructions to:

    a. Decrease his intake of eggs and whole milk products.
    b. Decrease the amount of glucose in his diet.
    c. Take cholinesterase as prescribed.
    d. Keep up the good work!

82. Quality improvement indicators for facilities for older adults need to monitor the following types of high-risk and problem-prone areas:

    a. Fall risk and body image
    b. Adverse effects of polypharmacy
    c. Fall risk, body image, and hydration status
    d. Hydration status, hip injuries, and hearing needs

83. The aging process increases the chance of older adults experiencing presbyopia, which causes difficulty focusing on near objects. This is due to:

    a. Inflammation of the cornea
    b. Trauma to the vitreous humor
    c. Pupil reaction time
    d. Loss of elasticity of the lens

84. Many older adults take NSAIDS for discomfort. It is extremely important to monitor the following system for serious side effects:

    a. Integumentary
    b. Neurological
    c. Reproductive
    d. Gastrointestinal

85. Some older adults have a higher frequency of developing GERD due to:

    a. Increased esophageal muscle spasticity
    b. Effects of multiple medications they take
    c. Incompetent lower esophageal sphincter
    d. Decrease in HCL secretion

86. If verbal statements provide information for advanced directives and are provided by the patient to the geriatric nurse, the best way to make sure they are followed is to:

    a. Tell them to as many people as possible.
    b. Check them with the family.
    c. Document them.
    d. Don't do anything because they may conflict with families' desires for patients at the end of life.

87. Despite improvements in the health care delivery system, older adults do not always receive health care because:

    a. They don't want it.
    b. They convince themselves they do not need it.
    c. They are afraid of the consequences of illness and treatment.
    d. They cannot afford it.

88. An 87-year-old man fell over a throw rug and experienced bruising, a large amount of swelling, and was unable to put his weight on his foot. After finding out from an X-ray that he had not fractured his foot, he was told he had:

   a. First-degree ankle sprain
   b. Second-degree ankle sprain
   c. Third-degree ankle sprain
   d. Fourth-degree ankle sprain

89. Due to aging changes in the immunologic system such as decreased cell functioning ability, older adults are at risk for:

   a. Infection
   b. Immunological mutation
   c. Thrombocytopenia
   d. Anemia

90. Mr. Ryan, 63 years old, has benign prostatic hyperplasia, so one would expect his prostate specific antigen to be:

   a. 2.05–2.66 ng/mL
   b. less than 10 ng/mL
   c. 2.56–3.90 ng/mL
   d. 1.5–4.0 ng/mL

91. The percentage of older adults in nursing homes who are in pain has been reported to be as high as:

   a. 10%
   b. 30%
   c. 50%
   d. 85%

92. The purpose of obtaining certification as a gerontological nurse is to:

   a. Establish a minimal level of professional competency.
   b. Recognize excellence in practice.
   c. Demonstrate advanced nursing practice level of competency.
   d. Identify one's readiness for RN licensure.

93. Mrs. Pipekettle, a 79-year-old woman, had a hysterectomy last night. She was transferred to your unit from recovery this morning and has been yelling and trying to remove her bandages all day. The reason for this is most likely:

   a. Dementia
   b. Delirium
   c. Depression
   d. Bipolar disease

94. Frequent dermatological lesions experienced by the elderly include:

   a. Cherry angiomas, senile lentigines (liver spots), and skin tags
   b. Lichen planus, acne, and pytiriasis rosa

    c. Warts, moles, and acne
    d. Melanoma, warts, and cherry angiomas

95. Living wills provide which information if a patient should experience a terminal condition or a permanent state of unconsciousness?

    a. Written information describing the patient's desires for life-sustaining treatment
    b. Names a person for making health care decisions on behalf of the patient
    c. Provides information for the distribution of the patient's financial assets
    d. Provides for terminal care at the end of life

96. It is difficult to perform a pelvic exam on some older women due to:

    a. Vaginal atrophy and dryness
    b. Introitus shrinkage
    c. Labia minora and majora stretching
    d. Vaginal canal elongation

97. An example of primary prevention is:

    a. Breast cancer screening
    b. Diabetes disease management
    c. Annual prostate specific antigen testing
    d. Smoking cessation

98. Risk factors for osteoporosis include all of the following, *except:*

    a. Active lifestyle
    b. Family history
    c. Early menopause
    d. Caucasian or Asian ancestry

99. Older adults with diabetes mellitus experience macrovascular and microvascular complications. Some of the microvascular complications include:

    a. Hypertension, stroke, and myocardial infarction
    b. Peripheral vascular disease, venous stasis, and amputation
    c. Renal dysfunction, neuropathy, and retinopathy
    d. Stroke, pulmonary embolism, and amputation

100. A 78-year-old nursing home resident is prescribed isoniazid for a positive purified protein test (+PPD). He is also given a prescription for vitamin B_6 to prevent:

    a. Uveitis
    b. Optic neuritis
    c. Meningitis
    d. Trigeminal neuralgia

101. The purpose of ethnogeriatrics is:

    a. Ignoring cultural practices because all people have basically the same needs
    b. Developing cultural competence in the care of older adults

c. Spending minimal time in the patient's room when there is a language barrier so as not to confuse the patient

d. Avoiding the use of an interpreter in order to help the patient learn a different language

102. New onset seizures can occur with young or older adults. With older adults the most frequent cause of seizures is:

a. Cerebrovascular disease
b. Pulmonary disease
c. Immunological deficiency
d. Electrolyte imbalance

103. The nurse discusses a core set of screening and assessment elements that form the foundation of the comprehensive assessment for all residents of long-term care facilities. This assessment tool is called the:

a. Minimum Data Set
b. OASIS
c. Resident Assessment Set
d. Maximum Dependency Scale

104. Professional nursing is best defined as:

a. Caring and nurturing
b. Safe and therapeutic
c. Holistic and caring
d. Organized and task oriented

105. Geriatric facilities should conduct quality improvement measurements on the following outcomes:

a. Medication errors, falls, skin breakdown, and infection rates
b. Rate of polypharmacy, incident report rate, and nurse satisfaction
c. Number of medications used per patient, infection rate, and falls
d. Falls, patient gender, and nurse education

106. Due to the increase in anterior-posterior diameter of the thorax from the aging process, one will typically elicit the following sound with percussion when assessing older adults:

a. Flat
b. Dull
c. Resonance
d. Hyperresonance

107. A 68-year-old woman presents for the third time after her annual physical exam with no complaints or symptoms but isolated systolic hypertension with a blood pressure of 156/78 on both arms and a similar repeat response within 30 minutes. She has followed a low-salt and low-fat diet appropriately and exercises for 30 minutes each day with no change in her blood pressure. The next step (not including pharmacological treatment) for her will be:

a. 24-hour ambulatory blood pressure monitoring
b. Admission to cardiac rehabilitation

    c. Admission to emergency department for malignant hypertension

    d. Blood work to determine her catecholamine response

108. First-line disease-modifying drugs for rheumatoid arthritis include:

    a. Tylenol, Aleve

    b. Percocet, phenobarbitol

    c. Methotrexate, hydroxychloroquine (Plaquenil)

    d. Elavil, Prozac

109. Four members of an assisted living facility's chess team complain of seeing colored rings around the lights and has been having a difficult time seeing the chess pieces and the board. This individual needs to see an ophthalmologist for:

    a. Astigmatism

    b. Macular degeneration

    c. Glaucoma

    d. Retinal detachment

110. Harriet Gray has developed a decubitus ulcer on her coccyx. All of the following risk factors may have caused this, *except:*

    a. Orthopnea

    b. Moisture

    c. Inactivity

    d. Shearing

111. When performing a functional assessment on an 82-year-old client with a recent stroke, which of the following questions would be most important to ask?

    a. Do you wear glasses?

    b. Do you have any thyroid medication?

    c. How many times a day do you have a bowel movement?

    d. Are you able to dress yourself?

112. The most commonly seen leukemia in older adults is:

    a. Acute lymphocytic leukemia

    b. Chronic lymphocytic leukemia

    c. Acute myelogenic leukemia

    d. Chronic lymphocytic leukemia

113. A research tool that has strong reliability indicates that it is able to:

    a. Measure an attribute consistently.

    b. Correlate the dependent variables with each other.

    c. Assess the participant's knowledge about a topic.

    d. Monitor how the environment is impacting the participants' responses.

114. Older individuals have decreased glomerular filtration rates generally indicated by creatinine clearance. This is measured by using the:

    a. Henderson-Hasselbach equation

    b. Tubular circulation formula

    c. Cockcroft-Gault equation

    d. Glomerular filtration volume

115. Which of the following are valid tools for assessing pain?

    a. SF-36 Short Form

    b. Faces Scale

    c. Geriatric Depression Scale

    d. Mini Mental Exam

116. Older adults are prone for the following side effect of opiates, tricyclic antidepressants, and anticholinergics:

    a. Diarrhea

    b. Abdominal cramping

    c. Muscular aches

    d. Constipation

117. The following age-related changes may affect older adults' ability to respond to cold temperatures

    a. Increased cardiac output

    b. Increased subcutaneous tissue

    c. Increased peripheral circulation

    d. Decreased muscle mass

118. An example of an outcomes audit would be:

    a. Testing the nurses regarding their knowledge of high-risk indicators

    b. Measuring the number of patients who had falls in their bedrooms

    c. Surveying the patients for their perceptions of how well the nurse administrator does his or her job

    d. Providing outcome data to the families regarding health care

119. Laurie Gunter is considered a pioneer of aging research for her work in the field of gerontological nursing during the:

    a. 1940s

    b. 1950s

    c. 1960s

    d. 1970s

120. Body mass index (BMI) is determined by calculating one's weight and height and using a BMI calculator wheel by plugging in the weight and height to determine BMI. A normal BMI for an older adult would be:

    a. 30 or higher

    b. 25 to 29.9

    c. 18.5 to 24.9

    d. Below 18.5

121. Infection is more difficult to assess in older adults because they tend to not be able to manifest the typical symptoms of infection, including:

    a. Fever and increased white blood cell count

    b. Increased red blood cells and increased platelets

    c. Fever and increased platelets

    d. Heat rash and tachypnea

122. Older adults have a decreased ability to respond to dim light due to decreased retinal illumination with aging. A good example of this is when an older adult goes into a dark movie theater after the movie has started. The person should be sure to:

    a. Take extra time to adapt to the dim light before trying to find a seat

    b. Get new prescriptive lenses to assist with the adaptation to darkness

    c. Never go alone to a dark setting

    d. Avoid darkened settings entirely

123. Spiritual care begins with:

    a. A plan of care

    b. Assessment

    c. Diagnosis of spiritual distress

    d. Discharge planning

124. The primary source of payment for older adult health care is:

    a. Medicare

    b. Medicaid

    c. Private insurance

    d. Medigap

125. Due to the physiological changes in the pulmonary system such as decreased vital capacity, decreased gas exchange, and decreased cough reflex, older postoperative patients are more likely to experience:

    a. Pulmonary embolus and pleuritis

    b. Pneumonia and atelectasis

    c. Pleural effusion and pneumothorax

    d. Bronchiectasis and rib fracture

126. Nurses must be aware of which of the following age-related changes that affect continence?

    a. An increase in the bladder capacity

    b. A decrease in bladder muscle tone, which results in a lessened ability to postpone voiding

    c. A decrease in residual volume to less than 20 mL

    d. An increased perception of the sensation of the urge to void

127. A 78-year-old man presents to the emergency department with a complaint of dizziness whenever he stands up. He has been diagnosed with benign prostate hyperplasia and has been taking doxazosin (Cardura) for approximately 2 weeks. Your priority action is to:

    a. Discuss time of administration with the patient.

    b. Perform orthostatic blood pressure and pulse assessment.

    c. Prepare him for intravenous hydration.

    d. Teach him the benefits of a low-sodium diet.

128. Approximately what percentage of hospice patients are considered older adults?

    a. 25%
    b. 50%
    c. 75%
    d. 100%

129. An example of a standard tool of assessment used frequently with older adults to plan high-quality care is:

    a. Medicaid survey
    b. Medicare assessment
    c. Older American Resources and Services Assessment
    d. Geriatric Activity Tool

130. Debilitated older adults who are bed- or chair-bound experience decubitus ulcers on their bony prominences more so than younger debilitated patients. The general sequence of manifestations is:

    a. Maceration of skin, edema, ulceration
    b. Macular rash, blistering, ulceration
    c. Ecchymosis, erythema, ulceration
    d. Erythema, edema, blistering, ulceration

131. An 88-year-old woman complains of shoulder pain that has been increasing over the last 6 months. She is assessed and diagnosed with impingement syndrome, which is most likely a result of:

    a. Frozen shoulder
    b. Wearing an arm sling for longer than 3 months
    c. Rotator cuff tendonitis
    d. Thoracic outlet syndrome

132. The following is a classical ethical principle often employed in gerontology:

    a. Malpractice
    b. Competency
    c. Beneficence
    d. Accountability

133. You are administering oral medications to a 70-year-old patient and he complains of sore lips and a burning sensation on his tongue and asks if he can get the medications in a different way. These symptoms are probably a manifestation of:

    a. Thallasemia
    b. Iron deficiency anemia
    c. Sideroblastic anemia
    d. Sickle cell disease

134. The most common type of hearing loss among older adults is:

    a. Presbycusis
    b. Lipidocusis

    c. Meniere's disease

    d. Arcus senilus

135. It is not uncommon for older adults to experience fecal incontinence caused by changes in the gastrointestinal system such as:

    a. Increased peristalsis

    b. Loss of sphincter control

    c. Increased tonicity of anal column

    d. Diverticulosis

136. A 65-year-old man has a history of using Percocet and NSAIDs for lower back pain; he drinks three beers daily and more on weekends. He notes that he is turning yellow, feels confused, is dizzy, and has no energy. When he notices that he has bright red blood in the toilet after a bowel movement, he presents at the emergency department. Your priority concern is:

    a. Referral to the transplant coordinator

    b. To stabilize his vital signs and give fluid resuscitation

    c. To assess his mental status to establish a baseline

    d. Pain management

137. Initial treatment for seizures in older adults includes:

    a. Cardiovascular stabilization

    b. Airway protection

    c. Keeping patient safe from harm

    d. Oxygen delivery

138. One of the greatest barriers to successful interventions to help problem older drinkers is that:

    a. Older adults don't usually drive, so intoxication while driving is not detected.

    b. Nurses and health care professionals fail to detect problem alcohol use.

    c. Many of the medications taken by older adults mimic the effects of alcohol.

    d. Alcoholism occurs so rarely in the elderly that interventions are usually not necessary.

139. The use of histamine H_2 blockers can cause problems with older adults due to drug interactions with the numerous medications they take and other central nervous system side effects. An example of these antihistamines is:

    a. Cimetadine (Tagamet)

    b. Clarithromycin (Biaxin)

    c. Raloxifene (Evista)

    d. Fexofenadine (Allegra)

140. Medicare and Medicaid legislation is important for all of the following reasons *except:*

    a. It provides health care coverage for the most vulnerable segments of U.S. society.

b. It was an initial step toward federal health care coverage.

c. It built upon the Social Security Act.

d. It was the first federal health care legislation to be broadly supported by the American Medical Association.

141. The increase in the older adult population will likely:

a. Stabilize in the future

b. Continue for some years to come

c. Stop by the year 2030

d. Be impossible to predict

142. A 77-year-old woman has been admitted for heart failure. You prepare her for a blood draw that includes CBC with differential and:

a. CA-125 and C-reactive protein

b. Brain natriuretic peptide and complete chemistry profile

c. ANA titer and electrolytes

d. CA-33 and complete chemistry profile

143. A 76-year-old diabetic woman has a hemoglobin A1c of 8.9, so she is going to be started on glargine (Lantus) insulin. Administration will be:

a. With three meals

b. Once a day

c. Before breakfast and dinner

d. At bedtime

144. Men experience andropause with the gradual decline in testosterone and other hormones as they age. Erectile dysfunction is not a normal part of the aging process but rather is due to conditions such as:

a. Immunological dysfunction

b. Cardiovascular dysfunction

c. Renal dysfunction

d. Dermatologic dysfunction

145. Many physiological changes occur with aging; however, it is a fairly individual process that depends on the following variables:

a. Gender, socioeconomic status, and genetic makeup

b. Genetic makeup, health behaviors, and availability of resources

c. Comorbidities, gender, and health behaviors

d. Availability of resources, socioeconomic status, and smoking history

146. Older adults have a high frequency of folic acid deficiency anemia, which is often the result of:

a. Poor nutrition

b. Genetic factors

c. Coagulopathy

d. Inflammation

147. A family caregiver has been caring for her elderly mother for several years. The caregiver is becoming very tired from the 24-hour-a-day responsibility of caring for her mother. The nurse would most likely suggest which of the following alternatives first?

    a. Acute care
    b. Hospice care
    c. Placing her mother in a nursing home
    d. Respite care

148. Regarding sexuality in older adults, nurses should know that:

    a. Sexuality is not an important part of older adult's lives.
    b. Impotency is a natural occurrence with age.
    c. A number of chronic illnesses affect the sexual function of the elderly.
    d. Men older than 75 years of age are incapable of fathering a child.

149. Health care institutions in some states must provide advance directives to their patients. This means that:

    a. The institution believes in euthanasia.
    b. The patients can declare their desires regarding end-of-life care.
    c. The patients will receive a full resuscitation if the situation requires it.
    d. No do-not-resuscitate decisions can be made.

150. Older adults with asthma frequently have viral infections prior to experiencing:

    a. Acute emphysema
    b. Pneumonia
    c. Acute exacerbations of their asthma
    d. Acute respiratory failure

151. A 70-year-old woman is being discharged to her home after being hospitalized for management of her bradycardia. She tells you that she has recently gained weight, lost all of her energy, always feels tired, and experiences general muscle aches and pains in her extremities. She tells you that the cardiologist is having her see her primary care provider for a work-up because they found some abnormal laboratory results regarding her thyroid. You are not surprised that she is diagnosed with:

    a. Hyperthyroidism
    b. Multinodular goiter
    c. Hypothyroidism
    d. Graves' disease

152. Ms. Zuniga, age 65, is worried about developing osteoporosis. Which of the following assessment findings would indicate that she may be at risk for osteoporosis?

    a. She exercises at least three times per week.
    b. She drinks three to four glasses of milk per day.

c. She is of Asian ethnicity.

d. She enjoys an occasional glass of wine.

153. An 87-year-old man asks you to explain what the action of losartin (Cozaar) is. Your explanation is that the drug:

a. Prevents high blood pressure

b. Promotes the excretion of potassium

c. Inhibits the conversion of angiotensin I to angiotensin II

d. Prevents the secretion of natriuretic peptide

154. It is imperative that health care providers ask older adults about common problems of aging, such as:

a. Financial resources, ability to communicate with neighbors, and musculoskeletal disorders

b. Depression, dementia, urinary function, and health literacy

c. Financial resources, urinary function, and history of drug abuse

d. Anxiety, depression, bipolar disorder, and schizophrenia

155. Normal changes of aging that affect older adults include which of the following?

a. Loss of teeth

b. Changes in senses of smell and taste

c. Loneliness and social isolation

d. All of the above

156. Mr. Foley, age 88, has lived with his son, daughter-in-law, and grandchildren for 5 years. He has recently been very afraid of the dark, the neighbors, and his grandchildren. He is afraid someone is trying to hurt him. This condition is most likely described as:

a. Depression

b. Paranoia

c. Amnesia

d. Memory loss

157. When older adults cannot afford health care, they often become _____ with treatment plans of care.

a. Angry

b. Noncompliant

c. Disgruntled

d. Frustrated

158. Religion is defined as:

a. A framework within which older adults search for meaning and purpose in life

b. An organized system of beliefs, practices, and rituals designed to foster closeness to a sacred reality

c. A means by which older adults complete developmental tasks of aging

d. A means by which older adults accomplish physical dimensions of aging

159. The nurses at a long-term care facility are having difficulty implementing a new wound procedure. Many of the nurses are unfamiliar with the procedure and are notifying you that they do not feel comfortable with performing the wound care. What would you do if you were the director of nursing?

    a. Ask the nurses to collaborate with each other regarding the new procedure.
    b. Have the medical director teach the nurses about the wound care.
    c. Have one nurse volunteer to develop and teach the wound care after learning it from a wound care consultant who is familiar with the procedure.
    d. Call another long-term care facility and ask how to perform the wound care.

160. When a medical diagnosis cannot be found for chronic malnutrition among older adults, nurses may consider the possibility of which syndrome?

    a. Polypharmacy
    b. Hypertension
    c. Failure to thrive
    d. Gall stones

161. It is not uncommon for older adults to experience systolic murmurs such as:

    a. Aortic stenosis
    b. Aortic regurgitation
    c. Mitral stenosis
    d. Systolic panmurmur

162. An 86-year-old man has scaly, horny lesions on his trunk. This is most likely:

    a. Contact dermatitis
    b. Seborrheic keratosis
    c. Actinic keratosis
    d. Lichen planus

163. A research tool that has strong reliability indicates that it is able to:

    a. Measure an attribute consistently.
    b. Correlate the dependent variables with each other.
    c. Assess the participant's knowledge about a topic.
    d. Monitor how the environment is impacting the participant's responses.

164. Cardiovascular changes with aging affect the endothelial walls of the vessels because of:

    a. Increased levels of collagen
    b. Increased elasticity
    c. Decreased levels of elastin
    d. Decreased levels of calcium

165. Many older women experience a connective tissue disorder that is associated with giant cell arteritis. This syndrome is:

   a. Temporal arteritis
   b. Polymyalgia rheumatica
   c. Rheumatoid arthritis
   d. Chronic fatigue syndrome

166. A newly diagnosed 66-year-old patient with type 2 diabetes mellitus asks why she has to take insulin when her friends take oral drugs for their diabetes. Her fasting blood sugar was 220 and she had been experiencing polydipsia, polyphagia, and polyuria. Your answer includes the following explanation:

   a. Insulin will provide the quickest way to reach the optimum glycemic target for you.
   b. The oral agents are far too dangerous because they cause cardiovascular problems.
   c. All new diabetics must go on insulin first until they are stabilized.
   d. Insulin may be able to cure diabetes for you.

167. An 86-year-old woman was admitted to the critical care unit after a fall that resulted in a subdural hematoma. The most important risk to watch for during her acute care hospital stay is:

   a. Changes in blood urea nitrogen (BUN) and creatinine, indicating renal failure
   b. Rise in triglyceride levels
   c. Effect of altered sensation on nutrition status
   d. Onset of delirium

168. The study of the actions and effects of drugs is:

   a. Pharmacokinetics
   b. Pharmacology
   c. Pharmacodynamics
   d. Pharmacogenomics

169. An older patient complains of sudden blindness in his left eye. He says he has severe myopia, wears his glasses, and has never experienced anything like this. He notes that he was golfing this morning and was riding in a golf cart over a very bumpy course. This is a vision-threatened situation requiring him immediately to be seen by an ophthalmologist because it is:

   a. Wet macular degeneration
   b. Detached retina
   c. Dry macular degeneration
   d. Acute angle glaucoma

170. Older adults have problems with urinary incontinence. The most frequent type of incontinence and most overlooked problems are:

   a. Urge and overflow
   b. Functional and stress

    c. Overflow and functional

    d. Urge and stress

171. A hallmark of palliative care is:

    a. Good environmental management

    b. Good anxiety management

    c. Good communication between the interdisciplinary team, patient, and family

    d. Encouragement of siblings to bring food to the patient

172. Pneumonia is a common reason for hospital admission for older adults. People with alcoholism, rusty sputum, and productive cough most likely will be diagnosed with:

    a. Streptococcus pneumoniae

    b. Haemophilus influenzae

    c. Staphylococcus aureus

    d. Klebsiella pneumoniae

173. In discussing sexually transmitted diseases with older adults, nurses should know that:

    a. Protection against STDs is not an important part of older adult's lives.

    b. Impotency is a natural occurrence with age.

    c. Condoms must be used to protect older adults against STDs.

    d. Men older than 75 years of age are incapable of fathering a child.

174. With aging, one has more opportunity to experience macular degeneration, which would cause:

    a. Floaters and blind spots

    b. Blurred vision and difficulty reading

    c. Blind spots and diplopia

    d. Trouble with night vision and astigmatism

175. When assessing laboratory results, a nurse sees that the blood cholesterol level of a newly admitted patient is over 240 mg/dL. This finding indicates that this patient has a:

    a. Desirable blood cholesterol level

    b. Borderline blood cholesterol level

    c. High blood cholesterol level

    d. Critical blood cholesterol level

176. A respiratory assessment of an older adult should include:

    a. Inspection, palpation, and auscultation

    b. Inspection and auscultation

    c. Inspection, palpation, percussion, and auscultation

    d. Palpation and auscultation

177. Because the presentation of an acute myocardial infarction in an older patient is atypical, it is important to monitor older patients carefully when they complain of:

    a. Shortness of breath, leg cramps, or headache
    b. Proximal extremity pain, dizziness, or chest pain
    c. Shortness of breath, fatigue, or epigastric discomfort
    d. Chest pain, headache, or tingling in proximal extremities

178. You are interviewing Mr. L, who has a hearing impairment; what techniques would be most beneficial in communicating with him?

    a. Request a sign language interpreter before you meet with Mr. L to facilitate the communication.
    b. Speak loudly and with exaggerated facial movements when talking with Mr. L, because this helps with lip reading.
    c. Avoid using facial and hand gestures, because most hearing impaired people find this degrading.
    d. Assess Mr. L's preferred method of communication.

179. Disengagement is an example of what type of theory of aging?

    a. Biological
    b. Sociological
    c. Psychological
    d. Moral/spiritual

180. A 66-year-old man with a history of alcohol and cigarette smoking is admitted for esophageal cancer management. He has signed advanced directives and has chosen palliative care treatment. He is experiencing:

    a. Dysphagia
    b. Dyspepsia
    c. Dysarthria
    d. Stomatitis

181. The Five Rights of Delegation was developed by the following nursing organization:

    a. American Nurses Association
    b. National League for Nursing
    c. American Association of Critical Care Nurses
    d. National Council of State Boards of Nursing

182. Sleep complaints among older adults commonly involve which of the following?

    a. Difficulty falling asleep
    b. Frequent nighttime awakenings
    c. Both a and b
    d. None of the above

183. An 86-year-old man was admitted to the critical care unit and is now exhibiting signs of delirium. It is important to explain to concerned family members that delirium _____ that is often caused by _____ in the hospitalized elderly.

   a. Is reversible/medications
   b. Is irreversible/Chronic Obstructive Pulmonary Disease
   c. Is part of the normal aging process/stress
   d. Develops over a long period of time/genetic factors

184. In gerontological nursing, all of the following are good examples of rehabilitative care, *except:*

   a. The process of assisting disabled persons to return to optimal health
   b. A specialized type of care that assists older adults to reach maximum functional capacity physically, mentally, and emotionally
   c. A type of care that restores the older person to a healthful state
   d. A low-level type of care in which the emphasis is on doing to the patient rather than working with the patient

185. Thinning of the subcutaneous tissue leads to increased skin injury in the elderly. Therefore, the most dangerous condition older adults are more prone to experiencing is:

   a. Hyperthermia
   b. Hypothermia
   c. Infection
   d. Inflammation

186. Because of the tendency among older adults to experience folic acid deficiency anemia, nurses need to teach older adults to eat a diet rich in:

   a. Salmon, tuna, and walnuts
   b. Nuts, liver, and green leafy vegetables
   c. Apples, pears, and strawberries
   d. Legumes, cereal, and dairy foods

187. A 68-year-old plumber presents to the emergency department with nociceptive pain secondary to myofascial pain syndrome. He thinks that the pain and stiffness he is experiencing may be due to overtime work. You are not surprised that he is given a prescription for:

   a. Tylenol
   b. Ibuprofen
   c. Codeine
   d. Percocet

188. To provide best-practice health care to older adults, it is necessary to assess and measure quality care indicators. Most institutions have the following committee to measure the data:

   a. Ethics
   b. Quality improvement

    c. Safety

    d. Risk monitoring

189. An 81-year-old man has recurrent arthritic inflammation of several pe- ripheral joints. He was diagnosed with gout 2 years ago and asks you to explain what causes this inflammation. You explain that:

    a. "When you have an infection, your body secretes uric acid, which trig- gers the inflammation."

    b. "Because you also have osteoarthritis, you are at risk for more inflam- mation from the joints, and this causes the gout."

    c. "You have excess uric acid, which creates deposits of urate crystals in the soft tissue surrounding your peripheral joints."

    d. "The inflammation is triggered by stress and alcohol."

190. Cognitive status needs to be assessed when older adults present with acute illnesses, because their cognitive ability may be temporarily af- fected by the illness. This acute change in cognitive status is termed:

    a. Dementia

    b. Confusion

    c. Delirium

    d. Agitation

191. A 78-year-old former stroke patient comes to the emergency department with new onset shortness of breath and a poor gag reflex. His wife is con- cerned that he may have aspirated, so he is admitted after the following assessment:

    a. Right-sided infiltrate after chest X-ray

    b. Bilateral rales auscultated

    c. Pleural friction rub auscultated

    d. Left-sided infiltrate after chest X-ray

192. Hemodynamic parameters such as the following are not affected by phys- iological changes of aging, even when exercising:

    a. Left ventricular thickening

    b. Cardiac output

    c. Systemic vascular resistance

    d. Preload

193. Physical restraints should only be used under the most severe circum- stances. If physical restraints are used, which of the following interven- tions are necessary?

    a. Check the restraints once every 8 hours.

    b. Keep restraints on a minimum of 3 days.

    c. Document why restraints are ordered, how they will be evaluated, and when they should be discontinued.

    d. Release the restraints at least every 4 hours, and move the restrained body part through full range of motion.

194. Which one of the following forms of health care financing is termed *welfare:*

    a. Medicare
    b. Medicaid
    c. Large group insurance
    d. COBRA

195. A 79-year-old woman returns to the nursing home with her daughter after attending a seafood chowder dinner. She complains of itching in her throat, a slightly swollen tongue, and mild shortness of breath. She is experiencing:

    a. Allergic rhinitis
    b. Drug interaction
    c. Anaphylaxis
    d. Cerebralvascular accident

196. Which of the following interventions would a nurse include in the care plan of a patient with a pressure ulcer?

    a. Apply pressure to boney prominences.
    b. Check areas at risk every 10 minutes.
    c. Avoid cushion devices that prevent pressure ulcers on the coccyx.
    d. Turn and reposition the patient every 1 to 2 hours.

197. A research tool that has validity indicates:

    a. A strong probability that it has been standardized in this country
    b. The tool measures what it is intended to measure
    c. The data have been randomly collected
    d. The findings are reliable

198. Nurses need to know that stress incontinence:

    a. Can be caused by bladder muscle weakness
    b. Is also called neurogenic bladder
    c. Is a leakage of urine resulting from weakened deltoid muscles
    d. Results in the total uncontrolled and continuous loss of urine

199. A 68-year-old man has been diagnosed with Parkinson's disease. He is on several medications to manage his movement disorder, which includes:

    a. Rigidity, bradykinesia, and tremors
    b. Tremors, incontinence, and aphasia
    c. Gait problems, salivation, and aphasia
    d. Seizures, rigidity, and balance

200. A 70-year-old woman has been diagnosed with acute coronary syndrome. She most likely experiences:

    a. Upper extremity pain when stressed
    b. Angina
    c. Neck, shoulder, and upper back weakness
    d. Chest fullness with stress

201. One of the attempts to cover the health care needs of U.S. citizens almost occurred as a result of which governmental act:

    a. Social Security Act
    b. Omnibus Budget Reconciliation Act
    c. Racketeer Influence Corrupt Organization Act
    d. Soldiers and Sailors Relief Act

202. Because many older adults tend to be malnourished, they have reduced albumin levels, which causes levels of free drug to:

    a. Decrease
    b. Bind to sodium
    c. Increase
    d. Bind to calcium

203. Physical changes in older women that affect sexual activity include:

    a. Enlargement of the breast
    b. Increased lubrication of the vaginal mucosa
    c. Increase in the production of estrogen
    d. Decrease in vaginal size

204. A 72-year-old man at the adult day care center where you work tells you that he has a dark mole on his back that appears to be growing. The best action would be to:

    a. Arrange an appointment for him to see the physician.
    b. Tell him to monitor the mole's growth rate for 5 to 6 months.
    c. Have him come to the center for a weekly check of the mole.
    d. Tell him not to worry, because most moles are not a serious medical condition.

205. Older adults are expected to represent what percentage of the population by the year 2030?

    a. 0%
    b. 13%
    c. 21%
    d. 45%

206. Older adults who experience urinary tract infections generally manifest the following as their initial symptom?

    a. Dysuria
    b. Pain in the pubic area
    c. Confusion
    d. Flank pain

207. An 82-year-old woman's husband has recently died, and she has been preparing to move from her home to her daughter's home. She notices she has a linear papular rash on the left side of her spine that is very painful. This is most likely:

    a. Herpes simplex 1 virus
    b. Herpes zoster

    c. Herpes simplex 2 virus

    d. Herpes virus 8

208. One reason for increased cardiovascular disease with aging is the presence of increased:

    a. Free radicals

    b. Cytokines

    c. Bradykinin

    d. Myocytes

209. Research on the causes of Alzheimer's disease is expanding greatly. However, currently, the only known risk factor for developing Alzheimer's disease is:

    a. Family history

    b. Possession of the trisomy 30 gene

    c. Herpes virus

    d. Viral encephalitis

210. Older adults experiencing infectious processes usually are monitored by their temperature changes and not their CBC with differential due to the fact that older adults tend to have:

    a. Little change in their segment and basophil cells

    b. No difference in neutrophil and eosinophil growth

    c. Minimal elevation in their white blood cell count

    d. A suppressed bone marrow response

211. An 82-year-old woman is diagnosed with glaucoma and prescribed timolol ophthalmic solution (Timoptic) 1 drop OD twice a day. She is already taking metoprolol (Toprol-XL) 100 mg every day for hypertension. It is important to emphasize that she should notify you if she experiences:

    a. Dizziness

    b. Headache

    c. Visual changes

    d. Weakness

212. Older adults have decreased tearing and have more chance of experiencing corneal ulceration. Generally, people with corneal ulcers complain of:

    a. Diplopia, sharp eye pain, and headache

    b. Bloodshot eye, photophobia, and irritation of eye

    c. Sharp eye pain, floaters, and swelling of conjunctiva

    d. Dull eye pain, headache, and photophobia

213. It is important for nurse managers to make decisions regarding health care delivery costs by using a:

    a. Cost-benefit analysis

    b. Mean ratio of what is necessary for best practice

    c. Cost utility analysis

    d. Cost effectiveness analysis

214. Restraints may be in all of the following forms, *except:*

   a. Side rails
   b. Vests
   c. Pharmacological
   d. Restorative

215. A 77-year-old man complains of watery eyes, postnasal drip, and itchy throat and ears. He says he just moved from the southern part of the country to a long-term care residence in the northern part of the country. He has had these symptoms since he moved in April and asks you what is causing his symptoms. Most likely, it is:

   a. Influenza
   b. Pneumonia
   c. Bronchitis
   d. Seasonal allergies

216. Due to decreased respiratory muscle strength and other changes of aging in the respiratory system, older adults with severe mucus plugging will require the following to remove secretions:

   a. Pulmonary angiography
   b. Bronchial biopsy
   c. Suctioning with continuous high-level vacuum pressure
   d. Bronchoscopy

217. The incidence of falls among older adults occurs most frequently in which environment of care?

   a. Home
   b. Nursing home or long-term care facility
   c. Adult day care
   d. Shopping malls

218. Mr. Brown, newly admitted to your nursing home, approaches you complaining of constipation. You explain to him that this occurs commonly in aging because of all of the following reasons, *except:*

   a. Lack of privacy
   b. Altered cognitive status
   c. Decreased bulk in the diet
   d. Decreased bowel peristalsis

219. Which symptom would be most characteristic of a urinary tract infection?

   a. Fever greater than 102°F
   b. Sharp pain in the abdomen
   c. Pain and discomfort when urinating
   d. Inability to void

220. An important factor to assess in the history-taking component of a physical exam is:

    a. Appointments the patient may have made at other medical facilities
    b. Drug allergies
    c. Whether the person has a pet
    d. Recent experience with fast food services

221. Due to the effect of inhibition of norepinephrine and serotonin reuptake by tramadol, it is not recommended for older adults who have a:

    a. History of seizures
    b. Concurrent use of steroids
    c. History of diabetes mellitus
    d. Concurrent use of diuretics

222. The presence of spiritual care at the end of life may provide relief from which of the following?

    a. Unemployment
    b. Pain
    c. Dementia
    d. Blood dyscrasias

223. An 81-year-old man has been experiencing epigastric pain after meals, bowel changes, and uncomfortable bloating. He is admitted to the hospital for treatment of:

    a. Gastritis
    b. Peptic ulcer
    c. Pancreatitis
    d. GERD

224. A 71-year-old woman has Parkinson's disease and is asking what the etiology of her illness is. You would include:

    a. Disorder of movement caused by cerebellar disease
    b. Disorder of the basal ganglia that decreases ability to initiate movement
    c. Brain disorder caused by aging that decreases beta cells
    d. Disorder of the pons that creates excessive cerebrospinal fluid in the brain

225. The young are considered to be younger than what age?

    a. 90
    b. 100
    c. 80
    d. 75

226. Neuropathic pain such as that experienced in postherpetic neuralgia is common among older adults. The following drug category is frequently used for treatment:

    a. Anticonvulsants
    b. SSRIs

    c. NSAIDs

    d. Acetaminophen (Tylenol)

227. There is a definite physiological change due to aging that affects gas exchange in the respiratory system, which causes:

    a. Increased carbon monoxide excretion

    b. Decreased carbon anion movement at the capillary membrane

    c. Decreased passage of oxygen from the alveoli to the blood

    d. Increased oxygen binding capacity for hemoglobin

228. The main function of a mentor for a professional nurse is to:

    a. Assist with career goal accomplishment.

    b. Work side by side with patient care.

    c. Become a good friend.

    d. Demonstrate complex clinical interventions.

229. A 78-year-old woman has Paget's disease, which is the second most prevalent bone disease after osteoporosis. She is most likely to experience some complications from the disease such as:

    a. Bowing of limbs, hearing loss, and arthritis

    b. Chest discomfort, loss of vision, and osteoporosis

    c. Neurological problems, liver failure, and tinnitus

    d. Renal dysfunction, liver failure, and arthritis

230. A 76-year-old man is admitted for rectal bleeding and open reduction internal fixation of his right ankle after falling due to an episode of dizziness. His hemoglobin is 10, and his hematocrit is 30. He denies taking any medications. He does say that he has had rectal bleeding on and off for several years and thinks he may have a hemorrhoid. An examination reveals multiple external hemorrhoids, and he is referred to gastroenterology. Initially, the plan includes:

    a. Stabilizing hemodynamics before surgery

    b. Application of Anusol cream to the rectal area three times a day and after each bowel movement

    c. Scheduling a colonoscopy immediately

    d. Showering four times per day

231. The scope of practice that a nurse can exercise is determined by the:

    a. State's Nurse Practice Act

    b. Federal government

    c. American Nurse's Association

    d. State government

232. A 66-year-old woman is admitted to the hospital for palpitations and tachycardia. She has a full battery of laboratory tests and is found to have a low thyroid-stimulating hormone level and a high T4 level, which indicates:

    a. Hypothyroidism

    b. Hyperthyroidism

c. Hashimoto's disease
d. Hyperparathyroidism

233. There are no physiological changes from aging regarding salivary gland function because there is:

a. Intact parasympathetic nerve function
b. A large secretory reserve in the main salivary glands
c. Increased tone of the muscular wall of salivary glands
d. An increased amount of neutralizing acid secretion

234. Sexuality is:

a. A continuing human need among older adults
b. Not necessary as people age
c. Too difficult for older adults
d. Only for the young

235. An 84-year-old man is visiting the clinic for an annual examination. The most important thing to include in your exam is:

a. CBC
b. Total cholesterol values
c. Vital signs
d. Cognitive status assessment

236. Many older people have itchy, dry skin. The best intervention to remedy this situation is to:

a. Use less soap since it is drying, keep well hydrated, apply emollient cream
b. Bathe more frequently, drink high-sodium beverages, use sunscreen
c. Keep well hydrated, take frequent oatmeal baths, apply mineral oil
d. Restrict time in sun, use sunscreen, wear light cotton clothing

237. Approximately what percentage of older adults are noncompliant with health care treatment plans?

a. 25%
b. 50%
c. 75%
d. 100%

238. Your 66-year-old patient has cauda equina syndrome and is complaining of the most frequently identified problem, which is:

a. Dehydration
b. Urinary retention
c. Tenderness in toes
d. Pins and needle sensation in toes

239. A 72-year-old woman is admitted with pedal edema, rales, shortness of breath, confusion, and recent weight gain. She has a history of well-controlled hypertension but no history of chest pain. She most likely will

be diagnosed with the leading reason for hospitalization for older adults, which is:

a. Hypertension
b. Heart failure
c. Coronary artery disease
d. Myocardial infarction

240. Mr. Jackson needs to leave his own home for an alternative residence. The reasons that older adults move from one environment to another include all of the following, *except:*

a. Increased income
b. Onset of illness
c. Change in family dynamics
d. Insufficient funds to maintain home

241. It is necessary to always be aware of the frequently experienced geriatric syndromes when assessing older adults in an acute care setting. These include:

a. Delirium, urinary incontinence, falls, injuries, aspiration, emboli, and risk of restraint use
b. Dementia, delirium, urinary incontinence, aspiration, and emboli
c. Urinary incontinence, falls, injuries, aspiration, emboli, and risk of restraint use
d. Delirium, urinary incontinence, skin ulcers, aspiration, emboli, and risk of restraint use

242. Gerotranscendance is an example of what type of theory of aging?

a. Biological
b. Sociological
c. Psychological
d. Moral/spiritual

243. Some older adults are maintained on theophylline-based medications for their chronic obstructive pulmonary disease. The theophylline drug level should be maintained between:

a. 30 and 40 ug/ml
b. 50 and 60 ug/ml
c. 75 and 85 ug/ml
d. 5 and 15 ug/ml

244. A few weeks after admission to a rehabilitation facility, Mr. Violet developed sudden onset cognitive changes. You would most likely suspect which of the following?

a. Urinary tract infection
b. Peripheral vascular disease
c. Malignant growth of a previously benign tumor
d. Gynecomastia

245. Decubitus ulcers generally occur over which part of the body?

    a. Spine
    b. Toes
    c. Bony prominences
    d. Knees

246. Aging increases the risk of having to undergo gallbladder surgery for stones because of:

    a. Widened bile duct
    b. Decreased gastrointestinal peristalsis
    c. Decreased pyloric sphincter motility
    d. Increased amount of bile

247. After an older adult falls, it is customary to perform an assessment that would include:

    a. Cognitive, psychological, and neurological assessments
    b. Focused physical exam and functional assessment
    c. Focused history and physical exam and review of functional ability and medications
    d. Incident report and notification of patient's lawyer

248. Due to the shrinking of the thymus gland with aging, older adults are more prone for infections due to:

    a. Increased hypersensitivity response
    b. T cell deficiencies
    c. Secondary antibody response
    d. Increase in antibody formation

249. Many older men experience fungal infection of their toenails. Symptoms such as thickened, distorted, and yellowish color indicate:

    a. Tinea pedis
    b. Tinea versicolor
    c. Onychomycosis
    d. Ballantitis

250. Regarding the sleep patterns of older adults, nurses should know that:

    a. Older adults are more tolerant to shifts in the sleep-wake cycle.
    b. Daytime napping of many older adults seems to compensate for night-time sleep disturbances.
    c. Rapid-eye-movement sleep increases with age.
    d. Older adults have a higher quality of sleep than younger adults.

251. In nursing research, a placebo intervention is generally used for the:

    a. Experimental group
    b. Control group
    c. Variant group
    d. Testing group

252. The following are the most common reasons that older adults do not comply with a prescribed drug regimen:

   a. Expectation that the problem is normal with aging, not wanting to bother anyone, high cost of drugs
   b. Fear of complications, anxiety toward swallowing pills, not wanting to take medications
   c. Religious reasons, preference for natural remedies, fear of complications
   d. Their caretakers tell them not to, religious reasons, anxiety toward swallowing pills

253. Lipid deposits in the eyes of some older adults are manifested by:

   a. A bluish circle on the aqueous humor
   b. A grayish arc surrounding the cornea
   c. Drusden bodies (yellow pigment) in the macula
   d. Cotton balls in the retina

254. Older adults have more difficulty compensating with their hematological system when experiencing acute or chronic illnesses such as:

   a. Infections and malignancies
   b. Pneumonia and neurological problems
   c. Musculoskeletal and integumentary problems
   d. Malignancies and hyperlipidemia

255. A type of healthcare insurance for older adults that is funded and regulated by the federal government is called:

   a. Medicare
   b. Medicaid
   c. Private insurance
   d. Medigap

256. Glomerular filtration decreases as a result of aging, and it can be further decreased by:

   a. Increased blood flow to the kidneys
   b. Some medications
   c. Penicillin sensitivity
   d. Stress

257. Older adults experience a decrease in taste sensation. Which of the following factors can further decrease taste?

   a. Diabetes, medications, dehydration
   b. Medications, fatigue, oral ulcers
   c. Infections, smoking, medications
   d. Medications, poor dentition, dehydration

258. As people age, they are more prone for developing a latex allergy if they:

   a. Have a high rate of exposure to latex, such as with frequent dental procedures or surgeries

b. Are more prone for hypersensitization responses
c. Have more immunogenicity
d. Have developed a compensatory mechanism to protect them from latex

259. What is the greatest risk factor for a fall?

a. Age
b. Cognitive impairment
c. Osteoporosis
d. Previous history of a fall

260. Gerontological nurses should advise patients with degenerative osteo-arthritis to:

a. Rest the involved joints as much as possible.
b. Apply ice to the painful joints.
c. Apply heat to the painful joints.
d. Exercise the involved joints regularly.

261. The Patient's Bill of Rights mandates that each patient in a long-term care facility or hospital has the right to:

a. Information disclosure, access to emergency services, and participation in treatment decisions
b. Access to their medications, dietary choice, and participation in treatment decisions
c. Information disclosure, the right to choose one's roommate, and a translator
d. A translator, access to emergency service, and dietary choice

262. A 68-year-old man has experienced GERD for many years and has managed it with daily omeprazole (Prilosec). He has a hiatal hernia repair, and his physician suggests that an additional test be done while he is hospitalized. This test most likely is to assess for:

a. Gastric acid contents
b. Intrinsic acid depletion
c. Helicobacter pylori
d. Diverticulosis

263. A 68-year-old patient is prediabetic with a fasting blood sugar of 108. As the visiting nurse performing his wound care, you teach him about how important which of the following activities are to promote his health and possibly prevent his being diagnosed with diabetes in the future?

a. Regular exercise every day, losing weight, stopping smoking
b. Taking insulin, eating a low-salt diet, stopping smoking
c. Avoiding stress, eating a diet high in omega fats
d. Joining a palliative care support group, eating a low-carbohydrate diet

264. When assessing an older adult's mobility and overall function, the Up and Go test is quite comprehensive and a normal result should only take about:

a. 2 minutes
b. 1 minute

    c. 30 seconds

    d. 10 seconds

265. Factors that impact sexual function among older adults include all the following, *except:*

    a. Medications

    b. Diseases

    c. Diminished desires that occur as part of the aging process

    d. Performance anxiety

266. A nursing home patient is complaining of increased thirst and a dry mouth. You are not surprised to see that she is on:

    a. Bupropion hydrochloride (Wellbutrin)

    b. Oxybutynin (Ditropan)

    c. Furosemide (Lasix)

    d. Spironolactone (Aldactone)

267. A 67-year-old woman has Raynaud's disease. She complains of cold fingers intermittently throughout the year. She has trouble doing her needlepoint and asks if there is any medication she can take to "warm up her fingers." Your response is:

    a. "There are vasodilators that could be used, but they may cause too much constriction in other vessels."

    b. "Have you tried wearing gloves when your fingers get cold?"

    c. "Let's discuss this with the physician next month when she comes for your physical exam."

    d. "There are medications that would dilate the small vessels in your hands and fingers, but these drugs would dilate other vessels, too, which could cause harm."

268. It is paramount to follow the Institute of Medicine's guidelines in order to improve:

    a. Staff retention

    b. The safety culture of the institution

    c. Medical and nursing malpractice insurance coverage

    d. Nurse satisfaction

269. A woman accompanies her mother to the clinic. She tells the nurse that her mother has been experiencing recent memory loss. The nurse should first assess the mother's:

    a. Cognitive status

    b. Dietary status

    c. Temperature

    d. Ability to ambulate

270. One rationale supporting the idea that aging causes people to become shorter is:

    a. Weakened vertebrae causing disk compression

    b. Osteopenia and osteoporosis

    c. Increased osteoclast activity
    d. Decreased estrogen levels

271. Older adults who are on long-term procainamide (Pronestyl) are at risk for developing antinuclear antibodies, which predispose the patient for:

    a. Rheumatoid arthritis
    b. Stevens-Johnson syndrome
    c. Seizures
    d. Lupus erythematosus

272. Mrs. Goldberg is nearing the end of her life and has ordered hospice care. The focus of hospice care is:

    a. Restorative
    b. Rehabilitative
    c. Palliative
    d. Curative

273. Older adults have a greater risk of developing insulin resistance and glucose intolerance because of:

    a. A redistribution of adipose tissue to the intra-abdominal region
    b. Decreased insulin release
    c. Increased C-reactive protein
    d. Increased antinuclear bodies

274. Your patient, 76 years old, is 2 days post-op ileostomy for colon cancer. He is going to begin chemotherapy and is getting prepared to be discharged. You know he needs more health teaching when he says:

    a. "I am going to have to adapt to this ostomy drainage since this is what I will have for the rest of my life."
    b. "I need to order some supplies for changing the drain bag so I will have them when I arrive home."
    c. "I am glad the chemotherapy will improve my prognosis."
    d. "I have an order for a stool softener to put in my ostomy bag."

275. There are multiple manifestations in postmenopausal women due to decreased estrogen, including:

    a. Decreased pH of Bartholin gland secretions
    b. Increased nipple pigmentation
    c. Decreased elasticity of vaginal epithelium
    d. No secretion of testosterone from ovaries

276. Advanced directives are designed to:

    a. Provide details about a patient's estate after death.
    b. Provide information on who should get the patient's car after death.
    c. Provide information on the patient's wishes after death.
    d. Provide information on a patient's wishes at the end of life.

277. The following agency accredits facilities such as long-term care agencies:

    a. Safety Coalition
    b. Joint Commission of Hospital Accrediting Organization
    c. The Joint Commission
    d. Older American Services Bureau

278. Which of the following assessment findings is most important to report when caring for an elderly patient with heart failure?

    a. The patient develops confusion or exhibits a change in mental status.
    b. The patient's blood pressure is 110/60.
    c. The patient's respiratory rate has increased to 28 per minute.
    d. The patient complains of a headache.

279. Good nutrition is an example of which type of prevention?

    a. Primary
    b. Secondary
    c. Tertiary
    d. Preventative

280. Your 76-year-old patient is admitted to the neurological unit with a subdural hematoma. You are not surprised to find out he had been in a car accident:

    a. 3 months ago
    b. 2 days ago
    c. 2 hours ago
    d. A few minutes ago

281. Hayflick theory is an example of what type of theory of aging?

    a. Biological
    b. Sociological
    c. Psychological
    d. Moral/spiritual

282. Successful nurse managers can use which type of conflict management to reach a win-win conclusion?

    a. Accommodation
    b. Compromise
    c. Avoidance
    d. Collaboration

283. An 81-year-old woman has her annual exam, and the blood work reveals increased serum iron ferritin, decreased iron, and decreased total iron binding capacity. You are not surprised, because this woman has the following treatment:

    a. Renal dialysis every other day
    b. Physical therapy daily
    c. Speech articulation therapy weekly
    d. Hydrotherapy for hips daily

284. Exacerbations of asthma are most frequently seen during the night due to:

    a. Fear of the dark
    b. Difficulty falling asleep
    c. Difficulty staying asleep
    d. Catecholamine surges impacting circadian rhythm

285. Most older adults with hypertension are not prescribed antihypertensive drugs from the following category because of decreased beta receptor sensitivity in the elderly:

    a. Calcium channel blockers
    b. Diuretics
    c. Beta blockers
    d. Alpha blockers

286. Autoimmunity is the leading cause of chronic illness that impacts women as they age. Which of the following is a systemic autoimmune syndrome that more women experience as they age?

    a. Degenerative osteoarthritis
    b. Lupus erythematous
    c. Rheumatoid arthritis
    d. Diabetes mellitus 1

287. What percentage of falls in older adults results in injury?

    a. 10%
    b. 20%
    c. 30%
    d. 40%

288. Which assessment tool has been used in assessing functional status in older adults?

    a. Beers Criteria
    b. Maslow Guidelines
    c. Katz Index
    d. Mini Mental Assessment

289. With orthostatic hypotension in older adults, it is important to assess for the following symptoms after a position change:

    a. Palpitations and headache
    b. Dizziness and palpitations
    c. Dizziness and lightheadedness
    d. Lightheadedness and palpitations

290. A type of healthcare insurance for older adults that is funded and regulated by the state government is called:

    a. Medicare
    b. Medicaid

c. Private insurance
d. Medigap

291. A 77-year-old man complains of not being able to hear well. He denies any problems with tinnitus or ear pain. He most likely is experiencing:

    a. Perforated tympanic membrane
    b. Otitis externa
    c. Otitis media
    d. Cerumen impaction

292. Which of the following joints endure the most impact from osteoarthritis and need to be assessed carefully?

    a. Ankles and fibulas
    b. Large toe and ankle joints
    c. Tibias and ankles
    d. Hips and knees

293. Many older adults experience problems with their feet due to poorly fitting shoes. The condition that results from pressure from a shoe rubbing against the bony areas of the toes is:

    a. Bunion
    b. Corn
    c. Hallux valgus
    d. Callus

294. A gerontological nurse is researching symptom management in palliative care for older adults in long-term care facilities. The purpose of the study is to collect specific information over a period of 6 months about medication interventions and patient symptom management. Which method of research should be used to collect data?

    a. Qualitative research
    b. Interviewing of patient families' perceptions
    c. Quantitative research
    d. Delphi survey

295. A 70-year-old woman complains of a lump on her neck in her thyroid gland. She is admitted to the hospital for diagnostic testing which will include:

    a. Fine needle biopsy
    b. X-ray of thyroid
    c. CT scan of neck
    d. MRI of upper body

296. Hospitals are required to:

    a. Write advanced directives on all patients.
    b. Make sure patients develop advanced directives before surgery.
    c. Provide patients the opportunity to develop advanced directives.
    d. File advance directives in medical records room immediately upon admission.

297. One of the main causes of delirium is:

   a. Age
   b. COPD
   c. Medications
   d. Participation in treatment decision making

298. Many older adults deny that they have pain and try to keep their routine without taking medications for pain. Using the following words may assist in more accurate pain assessment:

   a. Visual analogue scale of 1 to 10, asking them to point to their pain, asking them to explain their concerns
   b. Discomfort, hurting, aching
   c. Nociceptive pain, neuropathic pain, mixed pain sensation
   d. Autonomic, sympathetic, parasympathetic

299. You are assessing Mrs. L for a potential neurological disorder. Information that will help form a diagnosis includes all of the following, *except:*

   a. Results of the Mini Mental State Examination
   b. Cerebellar function
   c. Complete blood count
   d. Sensory assessment

300. Immunization is an example of which type of prevention?

   a. Primary
   b. Secondary
   c. Tertiary
   d. Preventative

301. Due to the aging process, it is not appropriate to use skin turgor as an indicator of fluid status; rather, one would use the following parameters with older patients to assess dehydration:

   a. Intake and output, mucous membrane moisture, and urine specific gravity
   b. Volume of respiratory secretions, intake and output, capillary refill
   c. Intake and output, mental status, and jugular venous distention
   d. Urine specific gravity, pulse, and intake and output

302. A 67-year-old man has erectile dysfunction and has begun to use sildenafil (Viagra). He and his wife were given specific instructions regarding the use of this phosphodiesterase inhibitor, which included:

   a. Taking it no more than three times in 24 hours
   b. Discontinuing its use if chest pain is experienced
   c. Taking it no more than once every 24 hours
   d. Taking it with grapefruit juice

303. Durable power of attorney provides which information if a patient should experience a terminal condition or a permanent state of unconsciousness?

   a. Written information describing desires for life-sustaining treatment
   b. Names a person for making health care decisions

    c. Provides information for the distribution of financial assets

    d. Provides for terminal care at the end of life

304. Mrs. B, 75 years old, is at your clinic for a preoperative interview. This interview may take longer than an interview with a younger patient because:

    a. As people age, they are unable to hear and thus interviewers need to repeat much more of what is said.

    b. Aged people lose much of their mental capacity and require more time to complete an interview.

    c. An aged person has a longer story to tell.

    d. An aged person is usually lonely and likes to have someone to talk to.

305. A 66-year-old woman had a right large toe bunionectomy yesterday, and she requests something for discomfort. Most likely she can have:

    a. NSAIDs

    b. Morphine sulfate

    c. Demerol

    d. Percocet

306. Self-actualization is an example of what type of theory of aging?

    a. Biological

    b. Sociological

    c. Psychological

    d. Moral/spiritual

307. As one ages, estrogen decreases and negatively influences bone growth by:

    a. Increasing osteoblast function

    b. Decreasing osteoblast function

    c. Decreasing osteoclast function

    d. Balancing calcitonin release

308. Immunosenescence refers to the aging of the immunological system and primarily affects the following in older adults:

    a. B cells

    b. CD_{12} cells

    c. T cells

    d. Hepatocyte cells

309. The prescription and administration of more medications than are clinically appropriate for an individual is often seen with older adults. This is called:

    a. Pharmacogenesis

    b. Drug toxicity

    c. Polypharmacy

    d. Overdose

310. What symptoms would be most characteristic of type 1 diabetes mellitus?

    a. Hyperglycemia, headache, sweating

    b. Excessive urination, high blood glucose levels, increased thirst

    c. Headache, hypoglycemia, tremors
    d. Low blood glucose levels, hot, dry skin

311. Due to a smaller number of functioning cilia and a less effective cough in older adults, there is more potential for acute respiratory infections to progress to:

    a. Pulmonary edema
    b. Pleural effusion
    c. Pneumonia
    d. Pneumothorax

312. An 84-year-old patient is experiencing cramp-like pain in his abdomen that awakens him from his sleep and is relieved with food ingestion. He says he has had this before for about 2 weeks at a time, and then it disappears. He most likely has:

    a. A gastric ulcer
    b. A duodenal ulcer
    c. Gastritis
    d. Crohn's disease

313. A woman has developed a decubitus ulcer on her coccyx. All of the following risk factors may have caused this, *except:*

    a. Orthopnea
    b. Moisture
    c. Inactivity
    d. Shearing

314. The nursing administration at a long-term care facility wants to assess patient and family perceptions of their facility's ability to manage patients' pain. They are interested in determining what the patients and families like about the current process and what they would like to change. To conduct this study, the following method of research should be used to collect data:

    a. Quantitative research
    b. Qualitative research
    c. Experimental research
    d. Gerontological standard survey

315. Problems with the U.S. health care system have stimulated many attempts at health care reform. Diagnostic related groups created in the 1980s attempted to correct which major problem of the health care delivery system?

    a. Poor care provided by hospitals
    b. Poor care provided by home care agencies
    c. Poor care in mental institutions
    d. Rising Medicare costs

316. Older adults experience decreased immunological function and are thought to be more at risk for the following:

    a. Thrombocytopenia
    b. Autoimmune disorders

    c. Eosinophelia

    d. Metabolic dysplasia

317. Due to the multiple side effects of various medications, most older adults have most effective pain relief from:

    a. Propoxyphene

    b. Acetaminophen (Tylenol)

    c. Meperidine (Demerol)

    d. Pentazocine

318. One of the elderly adults on your unit complains of dizziness, increased fatigue, and intermittent palpitations. He has several comorbidities but generally is able to participate in social activities. His laboratory work returns with the following diagnosis:

    a. Pernicious anemia

    b. Iron deficiency anemia

    c. G6PD anemia

    d. Sickle cell anemia

319. A new 80-year-old resident complains to you about her insomnia, waking up tired in the morning, and needing to nap during the day. After talking with her, you find that she has had trouble sleeping for the last 3 years, and the problem is no different now than it was before she came to the nursing home. A rationale for this sleep disturbance involves:

    a. Hypersecretion of the pituitary gland

    b. Hypothyroidism

    c. Modification of hypothalamic function

    d. Changes in cerebellar function

320. A treatment option for depression that blocks the reabsorption of serotonin is:

    a. Elavil

    b. Zoloft

    c. Haldol

    d. Restoril

321. A healthy older adult may manifest all the following changes in the respiratory system, *except:*

    a. Thoracic cage stiffening

    b. Decreased cough

    c. Fewer alveoli

    d. Fewer cilia

322. A 65-year-old man presents with complaints of getting up to go to the bathroom a lot during the night and being very hungry and thirsty. He has a family history of diabetes, and his fasting blood sugars range from 134 to 150. He has abdominal obesity, high lipids, hypertension, and weight gain. His symptoms suggest:

    a. Type 1 diabetic mellitus

    b. Type 2 diabetes mellitus

    c. Metabolic syndrome

    d. Syndrome Y

323. Prostate specific antigen (PSA) testing is an example of which type of prevention?

    a. Primary

    b. Secondary

    c. Tertiary

    d. Preventative

324. A few weeks after admission to a long-term care facility, an 84-year-old female developed sudden onset cognitive changes. You would most likely suspect which of the following?

    a. Urinary tract infection

    b. Peripheral vascular disease

    c. Malignant growth of a previously benign tumor

    d. Gynecomastia

325. HIV is an immunological syndrome that greatly reduces:

    a. Suppressor T cells

    b. Killer T cells

    c. Helper B cells

    d. Helper T cells

326. Activity theory is an example of what type of theory of aging?

    a. Biological

    b. Sociological

    c. Psychological

    d. Moral/spiritual

327. Which are some of the side effects of opioids that can impact the functional ability of older adults?

    a. Increased appetite, need for increased hydration, increased libido

    b. Gait disturbance, dizziness, impaired concentration

    c. Abdominal fullness, thirst, hunger

    d. Diarrhea, dry mouth, hunger

328. A 78-year-old woman has had trouble with tinnitus, interpreting sounds, and gradual hearing loss. This is most likely due to:

    a. Sensorineural hearing loss

    b. Meniere's disease

    c. Conductive hearing loss

    d. Sensorineural and conductive hearing loss

329. The hospice philosophy of care affirms patients' right to:

    a. Live and die with dignity

    b. Pain management while maintaining mental alertness

    c. A confusion-free end of life

    d. Spiritual wholeness

330. Benign prostatic hyperplasia occurs with approximately 50% of men by age 65. Common symptoms include:

    a. Flatus, abdominal distention, bladder fullness
    b. Polyuria, erectile dysfunction, increased frequency
    c. Dysuria, nocturia, bladder spasm
    d. Bladder fullness, dysuria, polyuria

331. It can be difficult to perform physical examinations of older adults for all of the following reasons, *except:*

    a. Polypharmacy
    b. Lack of standards
    c. Presbyopia
    d. Normal aging changes

332. Change theory recommends that nurse managers will be most successful in making a change if:

    a. The entire staff is involved in any decision making regarding the change.
    b. The nurses most interested in making the change are involved.
    c. Only the nurse manager controls the change implementation.
    d. The entire staff evaluates the outcomes of the change.

333. Long-term care insurance companies can best be described as:

    a. Acting in the best interest of clients
    b. Acting in the best interest of society
    c. Businesses
    d. A system negligent of profit margins

334. You are doing discharge health teaching with a patient, an 80-year-old man, who was hospitalized for diverticulitis. You will emphasize the need for a:

    a. High-fiber diet and prevention of constipation
    b. Low-fiber diet and fluid restriction
    c. Low-fiber diet and prevention of flatus
    d. High-fiber diet and prevention of diarrhea

335. Consequences of persistent pain with older adults include:

    a. Headache, metallic taste, abdominal fullness
    b. Lower extremity cramping, bladder fullness, infection
    c. Flat affect, diarrhea, spasticity of bowel
    d. Depression, anxiety, sleep disturbance

336. You are performing an eye assessment of an 80-year-old client. Which of the following findings is considered abnormal?

    a. Loss of outer hair on the eyebrows due to a decrease in the number of hair follicles
    b. The presence of arcus senilis seen around the cornea

    c. A decrease in tear production

    d. Unequal pupillary constriction in response to light

337. Nurse managers must be able to assess, analyze, plan, implement plans, and evaluate plans used on their unit and in their agency. This framework is the:

    a. Crisis Intervention Model

    b. Problem-solving process

    c. Decision-making process

    d. Nursing process

338. A 72-year-old woman has shingles and is expecting to have visitors today, among them her pregnant niece. She should be instructed to not have contact with the following individuals:

    a. Pregnant women, infants, people who are immunocompromised

    b. People who have diabetes, vaccinated school-age children, infants

    c. People who did not have chicken pox, older adults, people who have diabetes

    d. People with tuberculosis, mononucleosis, or liver failure

339. A 66-year-old woman admitted to the hospital for a sudden headache— "the worst headache of my life"—is diagnosed with a subarachnoid hemorrhage. Her manifestations would include:

    a. Headache, seizures, vomiting

    b. Seizures, change in sense of smell and taste

    c. Headache, stiff neck, hypotension

    d. Photophobia, headache, diplopia

340. Mrs. Jasmine is complaining of problems sleeping and requests a sleep agent. Which of the following medications would be unsafe to give her?

    a. Ambien

    b. Benadryl

    c. Halcion

    d. Midularium

341. Mrs. Carlson, a 73-year-old woman newly admitted to your nursing home, has a score on a geriatric depression scale indicating that she has depression. Your first line of treatment for her would be to:

    a. Refer her for psychotherapy.

    b. Recommend to her physician the need for immediate antidepressant medication.

    c. Do nothing, because this is a normal change of aging.

    d. Arrange a psychiatric consult for evaluation of her depression and treatment.

342. The hospice philosophy supports that dying is:

    a. Almost always preventable

    b. A natural extension of life

    c. Often associated with pain

    d. Often associated with delirium

343. Mr. Gray is a 75-year-old man admitted to your assisted living facility. In anticipating his care planning needs, you know that social role changes that occur commonly with aging include all of the following, *except:*

    a. Appointment of Social Security beneficiaries
    b. Onset of grandparenthood
    c. Retirement
    d. Grief over the death of a spouse

344. The nurse theorist associated with the concept of adaptation is:

    a. Sister Callista Roy
    b. Jean Watson
    c. Martha Rogers
    d. Imogene M. King

345. A 66-year-old man who is rehabilitating in the subacute unit of your institution complains of a lump that is movable and not tender in his axilla. He says he has had this lump for about 3 months, and it is getting bigger. It is most likely:

    a. A result of a virus
    b. Chronic myelogenic leukemia
    c. Hodgkin's disease
    d. Non-Hodgkin's disease

346. Cholesterol screening is an example of which type of prevention?

    a. Primary
    b. Secondary
    c. Tertiary
    d. Preventative

347. Practitioners who provide services to Medicare clients receive what percentage of the usual customary and reasonable rate of reimbursement?

    a. 20%
    b. 50%
    c. 80%
    d. 100%

348. Older adults are more prone to autoimmune diseases. A particular problem can occur with the thyroid gland with both a hyper- and hypothyroid manifestation. The hypothyroid autoimmune disease is:

    a. Graves' disease
    b. Thyroiditis
    c. Hashimoto's disease
    d. Multinodular thryoiditis

349. Older adults with systolic dysfunction have problems with:

    a. Fatigue
    b. Palpitations
    c. Venous stasis
    d. Chest pain

350. The inability of a caregiver to identify and provide for needs among older adults is classified as which type of elder mistreatment?

   a. Physical
   b. Psychological
   c. Active neglect
   d. Passive neglect

351. Older adults have altered pharmacokinetics due mostly to:

   a. Organ system degeneration
   b. Aging cells
   c. Increased sympathetic system uptake
   d. Release of bradykinin

352. A couple in their 80s have been experiencing problems tasting their food and request information regarding this. After giving them several ideas, you specifically mention alternatives to improve the following tastes, which particularly tend to decrease with aging:

   a. Salt and sugar
   b. All types of beef
   c. Lemon and other citrus fruits
   d. Tartness

353. An 88-year-old man complains of dizziness when getting into bed from his wheelchair and getting into his wheelchair from his bed. It is important for the nurse to assess for orthostatic hypotension on this patient. The nurse should test the man's:

   a. Blood pressure and pulse while lying, sitting, and standing
   b. Blood pressure while lying, sitting, and standing
   c. Blood pressure in his right and left arms while sitting
   d. Blood pressure upon awakening and immediately before he changes position

354. After hip replacement for a hip fracture, patients are taught to maintain abduction. Thus, these patients are told not to cross their legs because it may cause:

   a. Dislocation of the prosthesis
   b. Subluxation of the hip
   c. Incomplete dislocation of the joint
   d. Angular alignment

355. You are bathing an 80-year-old man and notice that his skin is wrinkled, thin, lax, and dry. This finding is related to which normal change of aging?

   a. Integumentary system changes
   b. Increases in elastin and subcutaneous fat
   c. An increase in the number of sweat and sebaceous glands
   d. Increased vascular flow to the skin

356. A 69-year-old woman with a 55-year history of smoking is admitted to the hospital for a work-up. She is concerned that she has lung cancer because she is experiencing:

    a. Shortness of breath, substernal chest pain, and cough
    b. Severe fatigue, left-sided paresis, and left-sided chest pain
    c. Shortness of breath, a change in her cough pattern, and fatigue
    d. Increased mucus, a hacking cough (especially when supine), and dyspnea

357. A geriatric nurse's work with dying clients ends when:

    a. The patient dies.
    b. The patient is in a pain-free state.
    c. The patient reaches self-actualization.
    d. The family's grieving process is complete.

358. Mr. Paul was admitted to your medical surgical unit after a radical prostatectomy. He has been yelling and trying to remove his IV. The reason for his behavior is most likely:

    a. Dementia
    b. Delirium
    c. Depression
    d. Bipolar disease

359. A 66-year-old woman has osteopenia. Which of the following drugs is likely to be prescribed to inhibit osteoclast activity and increase bone mass?

    a. Fluoride
    b. Risedronate (Actonel)
    c. Parathyroid hormone
    d. Estrogen replacement

360. For an elderly patient who was prescribed nitroglycerin to be left at the bedside for self-administration, it would be important for the nurse to assess the patient's:

    a. Vital signs
    b. Mental status for confusion or disorientation
    c. Ability to ambulate
    d. Past medical history

361. Orthostatic hypotension in older adults is diagnosed in which of the following situations?

    a. Systolic and diastolic blood pressure decreases of 10 mmHg after a position change
    b. Systolic blood pressure decrease of 20 mmHg and a diastolic blood pressure decrease of 10 mmHg after a position change
    c. Systolic and diastolic blood pressure decrease of 20 mmHg after a position change
    d. Systolic blood pressure decrease of 10 mmHg and diastolic blood pressure decrease of 20 mmHg after a position change

362. Gerontological nurses follow the Code of Ethics for Nurses in their daily practice. This Code was developed by the:

    a. National League of Nursing
    b. American Geriatrics Society
    c. American Nurses Association
    d. State Board of Nursing

363. As men age, they experience _____ in erectile function as part of the normal aging process.

    a. An increase
    b. An improvement
    c. A decline
    d. A loss

364. With the higher circulating levels of proinsulin and the less effective insulin receptor sites in older adults, there is an increased chance of insulin resistance as one ages. The following variables will further increase insulin resistance:

    a. Cardiovascular disease, NSAIDs, increased availability of insulin
    b. Alcohol, obesity, increased basal metabolic index
    c. NSAIDs, steroids, diuretics
    d. Sedentary lifestyle, incontinence, and alcohol

365. A healthy older adult may manifest all the following skin changes, *except:*

    a. Decrease and thinning of body hair
    b. Increased facial hair in women
    c. Fingernails becoming more brittle
    d. Balding in patches

366. A client at an adult day care center asked the nurse about the term *presbycusis.* The nurse told the client that presbycusis:

    a. Is a sensorineural hearing loss that usually occurs bilaterally
    b. Is a progressive conductive hearing loss that commonly occurs with age
    c. Affects more women than men
    d. Is a type of hearing loss related to the administration of medication that is toxic to the organs of hearing

367. An 83-year-old man was diagnosed with hiatal hernia. He had several symptoms similar to those caused by GERD, which included:

    a. Heartburn after a big meal or when lying supine
    b. Chest pain radiating to the left arm and shoulder
    c. Upper sternal pain immediately after a meal
    d. Right-sided chest pain on inspiration

368. Mr. Carter states that he is concerned because he notices a light-colored ring around the iris of his eye. What is the most appropriate response by the nurse?

    a. Tell Mr. Carter to talk to the physician about these types of concerns.
    b. Report this information to the charge nurse.

    c. Explain to Mr. Carter that this is a normal age-related change that occurs in the eye.

    d. Tell Mr. Carter that this condition could cause complications and must be monitored closely.

369. The most common type of incontinence that occurs with aging is _____ and is easily treated with _____.

    a. Overflow/bladder training
    b. Stress/Kegel exercises
    c. Transient/medication
    d. Urge/surgery

370. Geriatric nurses may best assist a grieving family by:

    a. Using an active listening approach to communication
    b. Stating that the patient died a "good death"
    c. Encouraging an expeditious burial
    d. Sharing in-depth details about his or her own experiences with a dying relative

371. Active listening incorporates several techniques, such as:

    a. Open questioning, accommodation, and collaboration
    b. Conflict management, acknowledging, and negotiating
    c. Open questioning, acknowledging, and summarizing
    d. Framing, grouping similar ideas, and accommodation

372. Lipid-soluble drugs have decreased plasma levels in older adults due to older adults':

    a. Increased body fat
    b. Increased lean mass
    c. Increased total body water
    d. Increased serum osmotic pressure

373. Who was the founder of hospice?

    a. Ada Sue Hinshaw
    b. Adelaide Nutting
    c. Victoria Champion
    d. Dame Cicely Saunders

374. The nurse theorist associated with the concept of self-care is:

    a. Florence Nightingale
    b. Virginia Henderson
    c. Martha Rogers
    d. Dorothy Orem

375. It is important to realize that older adults with acute respiratory failure present a challenge for health management due to their:

    a. Increased work of breathing, increased compliance, increased $PaCO_2$
    b. Lifelong smoking habit, cardiovascular disease, increased vital capacity

    c. Decreased respiratory muscle strength, decreased airway and lung compliance

    d. Increased vital capacity, comorbidities, decreased work of breathing

376. Neurological cell changes that occur with aging include a deposition of Lewy bodies that are linked with a specific type of

    a. Obesity

    b. Heart failure

    c. Dementia

    d. Depression

377. Speech pathology is an example of which type of prevention?

    a. Primary

    b. Secondary

    c. Tertiary

    d. Preventative

378. Testosterone gradually decreases in men as they age. The primary treatment for androgen deficiency is testosterone replacement. The target serum testosterone level is in the following range:

    a. 300–320 ng/dL

    b. 230–250 ng/dL

    c. 300–400 ng/dL

    d. 300–350 ng/dL

379. To foster transformational leadership, nurse managers should use the following skills with staff:

    a. Accommodation, collaboration, and mentoring

    b. Time management, mentoring, and role modeling

    c. Risk management, organization, and priority making

    d. Motivation, identification of staff feelings, and emotional self-management

380. Hospital insurance for Medicare recipients is funded under:

    a. Medicare Part A

    b. Medicaid Part A

    c. Medicare Part B

    d. Medicaid Part B

381. An age-related change of the musculoskeletal system is:

    a. Height decreases with age, and posture becomes straighter and more defined.

    b. The lengthening of the spinal column results in a dowager's hump.

    c. Muscle fibers shorten and increase in number.

    d. Bone reabsorption causes the bone to lose calcium and decreases the ability to produce material for the bone matrix.

382. Hematopoiesis is regulated by several cytokines that are thought to decrease with aging. There are also two cytokines that increase and inhibit hematopoiesis with aging; they are:

    a. Interleukin 6 and tumor necrosis factor alpha
    b. Complement 23 and interleukin 4
    c. Interleukin 8 and ANA bodies
    d. Tumor necrosis factor alpha and beta cells

383. There is an increase in the various forms of elder abuse and this is linked with an increase of older adults experiencing

    a. Posttraumatic stress disorder
    b. Obsessive–compulsive disorder
    c. Mania
    d. Schizophrenia

384. A 72-year-old man presented in the emergency department with left sternal pain radiating into his left shoulder whenever he moves his left arm. Pain developed over the past 3 days, after he had built a small fence in his yard. He denies palpitation, shortness of breath, or dyspnea on exertion. His laboratory parameters and electrocardiogram are within normal limits. His pain is most likely:

    a. Muscular pain from overuse
    b. Atypical chest pain
    c. Anginal equivalent
    d. Rotator cuff dislocation

385. Taking several medications is referred to as:

    a. Polypharmacy
    b. A drug idiosyncrasy
    c. Toxicity
    d. A cumulative drug effect

386. Nurses on a unit make it a priority to have their morning care and medications completed by 10:00 a.m. for all of their patients. The staff is task oriented and concentrates only on morning care and medications; they delay other patient concerns until after lunch. The nurse manager on this unit practices:

    a. Trait leadership
    b. Situational leadership
    c. Transformational leadership
    d. Transactional leadership

387. Regarding age-related changes associated with excretion, nurses should know that:

    a. Age does not affect the excretion of drugs to any appreciable degree.
    b. When the kidneys are not functioning properly, drugs tend to remain in the blood stream longer, increasing the risk of drug toxicity.

    c. Most drugs do not affect kidney functioning.

    d. The glomerular filtration rate in the kidneys increases with age, resulting in an increase in the excretion of drugs.

388. A 76-year-old man presents with controlled atrial fibrillation and unknown fever. The sedimentation rate was increased but no other abnormal results were obtained. When asked whether he had been taking any medications, he said that he had been taking Tylenol frequently for a headache, and he pointed to his right ear and forehead. He was diagnosed·with positive antineutrophilic cytoplasmic antibodies and started on prednisone with rapid relief of his headache. What most likely was his diagnosis?

    a. Migraine headache

    b. Temporal arteritis

    c. Tension headache

    d. Vasculitis

389. The ultimate goals of quality improvement programs in health care provide:

    a. Cost savings, patient satisfaction, and staff retention

    b. Optimal patient outcomes, access to services, and cost-effectiveness

    c. Family satisfaction, optimal patient outcomes, and new technology

    d. Patient satisfaction, access to services, and telehealth services

390. Hospice care may take place in which environment of care?

    a. Home

    b. Nursing home

    c. Hospital

    d. All of the above

391. Fungal infections of the toenails of older adults are most frequently due to:

    a. Tinea versicolor

    b. Onychomycosis

    c. Tinea capitus

    d. Impetigo

392. Which of the following is an age-related change that occurs in the gastrointestinal tract?

    a. Most people become edentulous (lose their teeth).

    b. There is a decreased incidence of hiatal hernia.

    c. There is an increased incidence of pertussis.

    d. The secretions of the salivary glands diminish.

393. The process by which a drug passes into the circulation for distribution throughout the body is called:

    a. Absorption

    b. Distribution

    c. Metabolism

    d. Excretion

394. A 76-year-old woman has been diagnosed with bilateral age-related macular degeneration. Her main complaint is:

    a. Peripheral vision loss

    b. Eye pain

    c. Central vision loss

    d. Blind spot

395. A 78-year-old diagnosed with myelodysplastic syndrome for the last 2 years is admitted to the hospital because he is experiencing pancytopenia. This indicates he has:

    a. Anemia, leukemia, and non-Hodgkin's lymphoma

    b. Neutropenia, tuberculosis, and lupus erythematosus

    c. Neutropenia, anemia, and thrombocytopenia

    d. Thrombocytopenia, iron loss, and uveitis

396. Your 70-year-old patient with Graves' disease is scheduled for radioactive iodine therapy. When you discuss the treatment with her, you are sure to include the following information:

    a. There is a very small amount of radioactivity emitted after treatment.

    b. The patient will need to be isolated for 7 days after treatment.

    c. The patient will need to take thyroid replacement therapy immediately after treatment.

    d. The patient's diet will be very restricted for 1 month after treatment.

397. A nurse assistant asks the nurse to explain the word *pharmacokinetics*. The nurse defines pharmacokinetics as:

    a. The action of drugs within the body

    b. The movement of drugs within the body

    c. The use of drugs within the body

    d. Treatment of disease with medications

398. One cannot live in the United States without hearing about rising health care costs. There are many causes for these rising costs. However, these costs are most directly related to which of the following?

    a. An increase in the number of newborn babies with heart disease

    b. Increased autoimmune diseases

    c. Improved development and access to diagnostic tests and technology

    d. The evolution of a national health care system

399. A 78-year-old woman has recently been diagnosed with chronic renal disease and is extremely fatigued. As the charge nurse, you communicate this to the medical director, who prescribes the following to assist in increasing red blood cells in the bone marrow:

    a. Ziagen (Avacavir)

    b. Stavudine (d4T)

    c. Erythropoietin (Epogen)

    d. Granulocytecolony–stimulating factor (Neupogen)

400. An admission nursing assessment of an older adult experiencing an acute event should include questions about:

    a. Relationships with extended family, even if the patient has not seen these family members for a long time

    b. The older adult's summer vacation plans

    c. Spiritual assessment

    d. The older adult's preferred type of reading material

401. What information obtained in the health history would most likely have contributed to an older adult's COPD?

    a. Smoking since the age of 18

    b. Weight loss of 20 pounds in the last 6 months

    c. Working for 6 months as a construction worker

    d. No participation in a regular exercise program for the last several years

402. Which of the following theorists focused specifically on the nurse-patient interaction?

    a. Brenner and Wrubel

    b. Hildegarde Peplau

    c. Madeleine Leininger

    d. Martha Rogers

403. The goal of nursing care at the end of life is to attain:

    a. Palliative care

    b. Good oral hygiene

    c. A "good death"

    d. As little pain as possible while maintaining alertness

404. A 76-year-old in a long-term care facility is working on a group quilting project. You notice she experiences tremors whenever she is sewing but no tremor when she is resting and waiting her turn. The tremor is most likely:

    a. Parkinsonian tremor

    b. Essential tremor

    c. Drug-induced tremor

    d. Vitamin deficiency tremor

405. A 67-year old man awakens with a very painful and swollen right large toe. His physician performs a needle aspirate and finds urate crystals. The man is diagnosed with:

    a. Gouty arthritis

    b. Rheumatoid arthritis

    c. Gout

    d. Infected insect bite

406. Many older adults with Alzheimer's disease use acetylcholinesterase inhibitors and the following drug, which helps to slow progression of the disease:

    a. Donepezil (Aricept)
    b. Galantamine (Reminyl)
    c. Tacrine (Cognex)
    d. Memantine (Namenda)

407. A 66-year-old woman takes an oral magnesium antacid regularly. Due to older adults' renal absorption, health teaching is necessary with this patient regarding the potential of getting:

    a. Hypokalemia
    b. Hypomagnesemia
    c. Hypermagnesemia
    d. Hypernatremia

408. The endocrine disease that is seen in both genders at a higher frequency than other adult-onset diseases is:

    a. Hyperthyroidism
    b. Hypothyroidism
    c. Hyperparathyroidism
    d. Hypothyroidism

409. Assessment of depression can be performed using a standardized tool specific for older adults called:

    a. The Geriatric Depression Scale
    b. Beck's Anxiety and Depression Tool
    c. The Elderly Assessment of Depression
    d. The Suicide Assessment for Elders

410. Due to the high potential for errors in health care delivery, it would be prudent to adopt a philosophy from business that increases the focus on quality improvement in long-term care facilities. The concept that focuses on decreasing error, waste, and redoing work is:

    a. Six Sigma
    b. Ombudsman Program
    c. Seven Interventions
    d. Geriatric Standard

411. Which of the following observations would a nurse expect to make in a patient with chronic obstructive pulmonary disease?

    a. The patient has difficulty seeing distant objects.
    b. The patient complains of joint pain.
    c. The patient has difficulty falling asleep.
    d. The patient becomes short of breath when ambulating to the bathroom.

412. Older adults are more prone to developing type 2 diabetes mellitus due to:

    a. Decreased glucose intolerance
    b. Decreased sensitivity to insulin
    c. Increased glucose production
    d. Decreased insulin resistance

413. The CAGE questionnaire is helpful in assessing:

    a. Readiness for smoking cessation
    b. Alcohol use
    c. Safe sex practices
    d. Amount of water drunk each day

414. After multiple admissions of patients to the nearby emergency depart-
    ment for worsening heart failure, the nurses at one long-term care facility
    decided to implement some new interventions to improve care for heart
    failure patients. They began by reviewing the literature regarding this
    topic and then adapted what they read. This type of research is termed:

    a. Evidence from the literature
    b. Evidence-based research
    c. Content learned from others
    d. Knowledge-based research

415. Mrs. Lyons, 76 years old, has end-stage renal disease and is experienc-
    ing severe fatigue, is retaining fluid, and recently broke her wrist. These
    symptoms are due to:

    a. Increased circulating protein
    b. Electrolyte imbalance
    c. Lack of neutrophils
    d. Decreased granulocytes

416. Many older adults take medications such as some of the statins, calcium
    channel blockers, and antiarrhythmics and also enjoy eating grapefruit. It
    is important to teach these patients to follow this guideline:

    a. Stop eating grapefruit and grapefruit juice.
    b. Take the medications 2 hours before eating grapefruit.
    c. Take the medications 2 hours after eating grapefruit.
    d. Eat grapefruit with the medications.

417. Due to pharmacokinetic changes in absorption, distribution, metabolism,
    and excretion of drugs with most older adults, there is increased:

    a. Metabolism of drugs
    b. Drug sensitivity
    c. Liver detoxification
    d. Renal filtration

418. Which of the following statements describe age-related changes that
    occur in the respiratory tract?

    a. The alveoli are engulfed in tiny capillaries through which carbon di-
       oxide and oxygen are exchanged.

b. The costal cartilages that connect the various parts of the thoracic cage become more rigid and stiff.
c. Residual volume decreases with age.
d. The action of the cilia increases with age, causing an increase in the amount of secretions.

419. The Joint Commission is the accrediting body for long-term care facilities. It is responsible for assessing whether an agency provides high-quality care and also monitors:

a. Patient dementia and confusion
b. Quality of nursing research conducted in the agency
c. Performance and continued improvement in care
d. Mortality and morbidity statistics

420. A 78-year-old man complains of a gradual inability to hear the television, conversational speech, and high-pitched sounds in both ears. This is a common finding in older adults due to:

a. Presbycusis
b. Meniere's disease
c. Vertigo
d. Tinnitus

421. The following is considered a normal finding in older adults and may result from increased resistance to ventricular filling during atrial contraction:

a. S_3
b. Splitting of diastolic sound
c. S_4
d. Atrial gallop

422. Older adults who are long-term care residents often exhibit atypical symptoms of pneumonia such as:

a. Chest discomfort, dyspnea, and sore throat
b. Sore throat, leg discomfort, and fever
c. Changes in behavior, fatigue, and loss of appetite
d. Confusion, dyspnea, and tinnitus

423. Your patient, who is 77 years old, has vitamin B_{12} deficiency, rheumatoid arthritis, and hypertension. She has recently been experiencing symptoms of hyperthyroidism, such as:

a. Tremor, palpitations, and proximal weakness
b. Decreased appetite, fatigue, and depression
c. Fatigue, low energy, and sadness
d. Palpitations, dyspnea, and weight gain

424. Which of the following is an age-related change that occurs in the cardiovascular system?

a. The mass of the SA node contains only about 30% pacemaker cells.
b. The blood flow to the coronaries increases.

c. The heart valves stiffen and become thicker.
d. Lipofuscin decreases in the aging heart.

425. A 76-year-old patient is cared for at home by her son and is extremely emaciated, confused, and bedridden. She has a stage II decubitus ulcer on her right buttock. She is incontinent of bowel and bladder. The patient was wearing an adult brief that was soaked in urine and had saturated the dressing to the ulcer. She has had the ulcer for 6 months and it appears to be improving. What are your plans?

a. Keep the wound open to air during the day and covered with wet to dry dressing at night, make sure her position and adult brief are changed frequently, discuss plans for nursing home placement.
b. Irrigate the wound with peroxide, rinse with water, pack wound with dressing change every 6 hours, make sure her position changes frequently, catheterize patient with Foley catheter.
c. Irrigate the wound with peroxide, rinse with water, pack wound with dressing change every 6 hours, insist on patient being transferred to nursing home, make sure she changes position every hour.
d. Keep the wound open to air during the day and covered with wet to dry dressing at night, catheterize every 6 hours, make sure she changes position every hour.

426. Which type of nursing theory is abstract and used to connect the four main concepts of nursing?

a. Nursing grand theory
b. Nursing conceptual model
c. Nursing middle range theory
d. Nursing design theory

427. Dimensions of end-of-life care include:

a. Physical
b. Neurological
c. Ecumenical
d. All of the above

428. A 68-year-old man who is HIV-positive has been experiencing a low-grade fever, has lost 10 pounds in 1 month, and has been sweating at night. He is told these are called B symptoms, which are associated with:

a. Chronic lymphocytic leukemia
b. Non-Hodgkin's disease
c. Hodgkin's disease
d. Myeloblastic dysplasia syndrome

429. You are providing a teaching program on dementia to a group of older adults at a senior center. One of the residents says that her mother had dementia and asks you if she is at higher risk. Your response to her would be:

a. No, there is no relationship between family history and dementia.
b. No, trisomy 21 is the only proven risk factor for developing dementia.

    c. Yes, there is a relationship between family history and dementia.

    d. Yes, but the herpes virus and viral encephalitis are greater risk factors.

430. A type of health care insurance available for purchase by older adults to help pay for health care needs not paid for by Medicare is:

    a. Medicare

    b. Medicaid

    c. Private insurance

    d. Medigap

431. The loss of subcutaneous tissue decreases the ability to sense coldness and predisposes elderly patients to:

    a. Infection

    b. Hypothermia

    c. Influenza

    d. Hypothyroidism

432. The rate of absorption of drugs in the elderly may be slowed due to:

    a. Decreased peristalsis

    b. Dehydration

    c. Delayed gastric emptying

    d. Increased gastric acidity

433. Certain drugs such as warfarin (Coumadin) and certain central nervous system depressants produce more intense effects in older adults than in younger people. This is due to the greater likelihood among older adults of:

    a. Increased total body water

    b. Increased receptor affinity

    c. Increased catecholamine surge

    d. Decreased neurotransmitter connections

434. Ways to encourage adherence with a treatment regimen include all of the following, *except:*

    a. Patient education

    b. Encouraging a good relationship between the patient and the health care provider

    c. Encouraging the use of complementary disease therapies

    d. Simplifying the regimen to the greatest extent possible

435. A 78-year-old man has a bladder scan, which finds a residual of 60 ml after urinating. The average postvoid residual urine increases for older adults and falls between:

    a. 25 and 50 ml

    b. 75 and 100 ml

    c. 10 and 25 ml

    d. 50 and 100 ml

436. An 81-year-old woman complains of dizziness, nausea, presyncope, and problems with balance. After being worked up for the dizziness, the diagnosis given is:

    a. Meniere's disease
    b. Seizure disorder
    c. Benign paroxysmal positional vertigo
    d. Cluster headache

437. An 81-year-old woman is complaining of ulcerations in her mouth that are affecting her eating habits and causing severe pain. As the nurse manager of the unit, you are not surprised to see that she is on the following medication:

    a. Rosiglitazone (Avandia)
    b. Prednisone
    c. Alendronate (Fosamax)
    d. Furosemide (Lasix)

438. The role of the nurse manager includes:

    a. Carrying out the nursing process with each patient who has more than two comorbidities
    b. Following the organization's policies and procedures to generate high-quality care
    c. Meeting with the risk manager to determine the best possible insurance coverage for patients with disability
    d. Procuring funds from philanthropists for the unit's operating budget

439. Patient-centered care is described as part of the mission of most long-term care facilities. Some characteristics of being patient centered include:

    a. Nurse-driven, task oriented, and cost-effective
    b. Shared knowledge with patient, anticipated patient needs, and customized care
    c. Centralized, standardized, and specialty focused
    d. Time and task oriented and specialty focused

440. A 67-year-old woman comes to the nursing home's wellness clinic with a blood pressure of 155/98, abdominal obesity, total cholesterol of 266, and a fasting blood sugar of 130. After measuring her weight and height, you are not surprised to determine her BMI to be 33. She most likely will be diagnosed with:

    a. Cushing's syndrome
    b. Morbid obesity
    c. Metabolic syndrome
    d. Syndrome XI

441. The inflicting of pain or injury among older adults is classified as which type of elder mistreatment?

    a. Physical
    b. Psychological

    c. Active neglect
    d. Passive neglect

442. Regarding stress incontinence, nurses should know that this type of incontinence:

    a. Can be caused by bladder muscle weakness
    b. Is also called neurogenic bladder
    c. Is a leakage of urine resulting from weakened deltoid muscles
    d. Results in the total uncontrolled and continuous loss of urine

443. A 78-year-old presents with new onset of seizures to the emergency department. His wife reports that he has had difficulty remembering and making decisions and that he has experienced mood changes over the past 2 to 3 months. His diagnostic tests reveal:

    a. Cerebrovascular accident
    b. Medication interaction
    c. Brain tumor
    d. Meningitis

444. The geriatric nurse caring for a patient at the end of life knows that:

    a. Most older adult patients have resolved all their psychological issues by the time death approaches.
    b. Most older adult patients have accomplished all developmental tasks of aging by the time death approaches.
    c. End-of-life care often provides an opportunity to help patients complete important psychological and developmental tasks of aging.
    d. Discussing unresolved psychological and developmental issues is not appropriate in the nurse-patient relationship.

445. Sleep apnea is frequently seen in geriatric clients and is correlated with other chronic illnesses. Risk factors for sleep apnea include:

    a. Male gender, COPD, older than 75 yrs
    b. Male gender, obesity, older than 65 yrs
    c. Female gender, diabetes mellitus, obesity
    d. Female gender, emphysema, heart failure

446. Medicare Managed Care facilitated health care receipt by older adults through which mechanism?

    a. PPOs
    b. Free clinics
    c. State-run clinics
    d. HMOs

447. Many older adults experience constipation due to medications and inactivity. Suggestions for promoting improved bowel health include:

    a. Frequent enemas, suppositories, and fleets
    b. Exercise routines, liquid protein diets
    c. High bulk in diet, exercise routines
    d. Fluid restriction, low fiber in diet

448. Mrs. George is an 84-year-old woman newly admitted to your adult day care center with a low score on the Mini Mental State Examination. Your first line of treatment for her would be to:

a. Refer her for comprehensive geriatric services.
b. Rule out delirium and depression as contributors to altered cognitive function.
c. Do nothing, because cognitive dysfunction is a normal change of aging.
d. Recommend to the physician the administration of Aricept.

449. The following are leadership roles that gerontological staff nurses need to assume:

a. Communicator, visionary role model, and change maker
b. Fiscal manager, palliative care director, and staff development coordinator
c. Staff development coordinator, motivator, and risk manager
d. Resource manager, supervisor, and communicator

450. The number of annual elder abuse cases is estimated to exceed:

a. 200,000
b. 500,000
c. 1,000,000
d. 10,000,000

451. Immobility and having a prothrombotic condition secondary to cardio-vascular disease make older adults vulnerable to developing:

a. Pulmonary fibrosis
b. Deep vein thrombosis
c. Lupus erythematosus
d. Raynaud's disease

452. An 82-year-old presents with loss of night vision to the point that he feels he should no longer drive at night. He says "everything seems fuzzy." He most likely will be diagnosed with:

a. Glaucoma
b. Macular degeneration
c. Astigmatism
d. Cataract

453. One of the most significant reasons for older adults to experience adverse drug effects is:

a. Polypharmacy
b. Increased hydration level
c. Decreased fat tissue
d. Decreased lean body mass

454. Nurses must be aware of the following age-related changes that affect continence:

a. There is an increase in the bladder capacity.

    b. A decrease in bladder muscle tone results in a lessened ability to post-pone voiding.

    c. Residual volume decreases to less than 20 mL.

    d. There is an increased perception of the sensation of the urge to void.

455. Observation of posture is a key component of the following body system examination:

    a. Skin

    b. Cardiovascular

    c. Abdominal

    d. Respiratory

456. Older adults with long-term hypothyroidism taking levothyroxine (Synthroid) are at high risk to develop:

    a. Coagulopathies

    b. Bradycardia

    c. Anxiety

    d. Osteoporosis

457. A 71-year-old woman complains of ecchymosis, fatigue, and frequent respiratory infections. The physician orders a CBC with differential, and the diagnosis of leukemia is made. She remembers that her 83-year-old sister also has leukemia. Which is most likely her diagnosis?

    a. Acute lymphocytic leukemia

    b. Acute myelogenous leukemia

    c. Chronic myelogenous leukemia

    d. Chronic lymphocytic leukemia

458. Which of the following testing instruments is used to evaluate orientation, recall, and calculation?

    a. Beck Depression Inventory

    b. Barthel Functional Index

    c. PULSES Profile

    d. Folstein Mini-Mental State Examination

459. One of the residents of an assisted living facility is inquiring how to submit a complaint regarding the living arrangements. Who would be best for him to contact?

    a. Ombudsman

    b. Staff nurse

    c. Facility administrator

    d. Manager of grounds keeping

460. What demographic trend(s) are important to nursing during the next decade?

    a. Aging population

    b. Cultural diversity

    c. Poverty

    d. All of the above

461. Coupled with decreased liver and kidney function, older adults also experience the following related to their adrenal gland function

a. Increased release of mineralcorticoid response
b. Increased metabolic clearance of cortisol
c. Decreased metabolic clearance of cortisol
d. Increased functioning of the adrenal cortex

462. The withholding of necessities among older adults is classified as which type of elder mistreatment?

a. Physical
b. Psychological
c. Active neglect
d. Passive neglect

463. The end of life is often associated with which of the following physical symptoms among older adults?

a. Anxiety
b. Agitation
c. Depression
d. Pain

464. A 87-year-old patient in a long-term care facility has just received his first influenza vaccine. He experiences a moderate hypersensitivity response but does fine with an antihistamine. His daughter explains that he has multiple food allergies. He was most likely allergic to the following in the influenza vaccine:

a. Preservative
b. Egg albumin
c. Legume extract
d. Peanut oil

465. An 83-year-old woman has enjoyed summering at the beach her entire life. She has noticed several hyperpigmented macular lesions over the last 10 years but is most concerned when she notes a rough papular area on her right wrist. This papule is most likely:

a. Lentigine
b. Seborrheic keratosis
c. Actinic keratosis
d. Acrochordons

466. Nurses at a long-term care facility requested professional development on leadership. The nurse manager should do which of the following to fulfill this need?

a. Teach the nurses about the leadership skills that will help them become nurse managers.
b. Have the administrator of the facility teach the nurses what he or she learned in his or her business program.

c. Perform a needs survey of the staff to determine what they want to gain regarding leadership skills.

d. Tell the staff they do not need leadership development unless they want to be a nurse manager.

467. Which of the following is the *most* important use of the information obtained from the functional assessment?

a. Providing data to develop a medication administration record
b. Identifying specific self-care deficits
c. Classifying patient anxiety levels
d. Determining the cause of the disease process

468. Older adults with type 2 diabetes mellitus who have renal insufficiency should not be prescribed:

a. Pioglitazone (Actos)
b. Rosiglitazone (Avandia)
c. Metformin (Glucophage)
d. Insulin (Lantus)

469. With older adults, many drugs' half-lives are increased due to:

a. Coagulopathy
b. Decreased liver function
c. Increased liver function
d. Increased total body water

470. A 71-year-old woman has just had her annual gynecological exam and is surprised to find out that she has bacterial vaginosis. She is sexually active with her husband and says she has noticed a slight odor but did not realize it was abnormal. She has recently finished an antibiotic for an upper respiratory infection. Because of her age, she is more susceptible to infections due to:

a. Her active sex life
b. Decreased estrogen
c. Increased pH
d. Vaginal epithelium atrophy

471. The largest source of funding for health care services for the indigent population in the United States is:

a. Medicare
b. Medicaid
c. Private insurance
d. Medigap

472. It is important to assess older adults taking diuretics for symptoms of urinary incontinence such as:

a. Dysuria, nocturia, and anuria
b. Anuria, malodorous urine, and cloudy urine

  c. Urinary frequency, urgency, and nocturia
  d. Dysuria, polyuria, and cloudy urine

473. Older adults normally have a PaO_2 lower than younger adults. The normal range of oxygen for older adults is:

  a. 80 to 89 mmHg
  b. 70 to 75 mmHg
  c. 85 to 90 mmHg
  d. 90 to 95 mmHg

474. An effective means of nutritional assessment is:

  a. 24-hour recall
  b. Forced hydration
  c. Food guide pyramid
  d. Tube feedings

475. Delirium:

  a. Is reversible
  b. Is irreversible
  c. Is part of the normal aging process
  d. Develops over a long period of time

476. A 71-year-old presents to the emergency department with pain around his left ear, decreased ability to chew, and drooping on the left side of this lip. He is diagnosed with a condition that causes paralysis of the facial nerve called:

  a. Bell's Palsy
  b. Trigeminal neuralgia
  c. Herpes zoster
  d. CVA

477. Many unsuccessful nurse managers have authority as identified in their job description, but, because their authority is not linked with the following characteristic, they are unable to lead their unit successfully:

  a. Power
  b. Common sense
  c. Time management ability
  d. Organizational skills

478. More than one-half of all people older than 65 years have cataracts. Their most common complaints include:

  a. Strabismus and diplopia
  b. Blurred vision and night vision loss
  c. Diplopia and loss of color perception
  d. Blindness and floaters

479. Inflammation and infection of the gums and oral soft tissue due to build-up of bacterial plaque causes

  a. Stomatitis
  b. Periodontitis

c. Gingiosis

d. Alchalasia

480. Many older adults are diagnosed with prediabetes and type 2 diabetes mellitus. They are generally prescribed a drug that decreases appetite and causes weight loss. That drug is:

a. Metformin (Glucophage)

b. Pioglitazone (Actos)

c. Insulin glargine (Lantus)

d. Insulin aspart (Novolog)

481. Older adults who have anxiety disorders are often prescribed selective serotonin reuptake inhibitors (SSRIs) at a lower dose than what is used with depression. An SSRI that is used with older adults is:

a. Paroxetine

b. Fluoxetine (Prozac)

c. Buspirone

d. Ritalin

482. An 88-year-old patient often complains of leg cramping that is very painful when he walks but says he has no pain in his legs at rest. He is most likely experiencing:

a. Venous insufficiency

b. Restless leg syndrome

c. Intermittent claudication

d. Calcificanosis

483. The inflicting of mental anguish among older adults is classified as which type of elder mistreatment?

a. Physical

b. Psychological

c. Active neglect

d. Passive neglect

484. A 78-year-old man is admitted to the long-term care residence with Alzheimer's disease. He is in the final stages of the disease and exhibits the following symptoms:

a. Short-term memory loss, headaches, and hearing loss

b. Memory loss, mood changes, changes in personality

c. Headaches, long-term memory loss, incontinence

d. Memory loss, vision loss, behavior changes

485. Which dimension of care is most often ignored in end-of-life care plans for older adults?

a. Physical

b. Spiritual

c. Psychological

d. Social

486. It is significant to observe all patients who have diabetes for signs and symptoms of hypoglycemia, especially when they may have the flu or be dehydrated. These signs and symptoms include:

a. Confusion, tremors, weakness, diaphoresis
b. Irritability, hunger, thirst, hearing dysfunction
c. Diaphoresis, thirst, seizures, behavioral changes
d. Dementia, rash, chest discomfort, headache

487. The Balanced Budget act of 1997 had which main effect on reimbursement of care for older adults?

a. Changed Medicare from being a private insurer to managed care
b. Restored funds for Medicare
c. Restored funds for Social Security
d. Transferred funds from Social Security to Medicare

488. When assessing an older adult's ability to function with activities of daily living, it is essential that the interviewer be consistent in assessing for:

a. Either performance or capacity
b. The best possible performance of the individual
c. The individual's ability to function without medications
d. The individual's ability to function without assistive devices

489. In discussing a functional assessment during a team conference, which of the following statements would the nurse most likely make?

a. A functional assessment is used to evaluate the overall ability of older adults to independently complete their activities of daily living.
b. The major emphasis of a functional assessment is on the psychosocial well-being.
c. A functional assessment is not necessary until the older adult becomes familiar with the environment.
d. Many times, the functional assessment can be delegated to a nursing assistant.

490. Gerontological staff nurses will be more effective in delivering care if they develop teams to provide patient care. Members of the teams must include:

a. Registered nurses, licensed practical nurses, and unlicensed assistive personnel
b. A psychologist and licensed practical nurses
c. Pharmacists and occupational therapists
d. Physical therapists and recreational therapists

491. The most common type of bone fracture with the highest rate of complications in older adults is:

a. Wrist
b. Femur
c. Humerus
d. Hip

492. Which of the following theorists focused on caring as the central essence of nursing?

    a. Brenner and Wrubel
    b. Hildegarde Peplau
    c. Madeleine Leininger
    d. Martha Rogers

493. A 77-year-old nursing home resident is complaining of a tingling and very painful rash on the left side only in the mid-scapular area of his back. He is diagnosed with herpes zoster and is put on an antiviral drug. He still complains of the pain so you notify the physician, who prescribes the following:

    a. Acetaminophen (Tylenol)
    b. Amitriptyline (Elavil)
    c. Prednisone
    d. Fexofenadine (Allegra)

494. As men age they experience several physiologic changes such as decreased testosterone, which causes the following anatomical change in their uro-genital area:

    a. Prostate gland hypertrophy
    b. Prostate gland shrinking
    c. Scrotal tissue atrophy
    d. Testicular gland hypertrophy

495. Alcohol use is difficult to assess in older adults because:

    a. Older adults rarely use alcohol.
    b. Older adults are not usually in the workplace.
    c. Symptoms of alcohol use are consistent with dementia.
    d. Both b and c.

496. You have been asked to give a health teaching program on best dietary practices with iron deficiency anemia. You will discuss appropriate foods, which are:

    a. Fruit plate, milk, and vegetable tray
    b. Liver and onions, potatoes, and green leafy salad
    c. Legumes, yogurt, and milk
    d. Roast beef, peanut butter sandwiches, and spinach salad

497. Which statement most adequately describes the spiritual needs of older adults at the end of life?

    a. Spirituality may provide a framework within which older adults search for meaning and purpose in life.
    b. Pain management at the end of life is more important than attention to spiritual needs.
    c. Accomplishing developmental and psychological tasks at the end of life is more important than accomplishing spiritual tasks.

d. Replacing dying older adults at their workplace is more important than helping them address spiritual needs at the end of life.

498. A 77-year-old woman has a long history of estrogen replacement therapy and hypertension. She presents with dysarthria, left-sided hemiplegia, and diminished gag reflex. The etiology of these symptoms is:

   a. Transient ischemic attack
   b. Thrombotic cerebrovascular accident
   c. Hemorrhagic cerebrovascular accident
   d. Brain tumor

499. The RN team leader on a long-term care geriatric unit of 44 patients will be responsible for 22 of them. Most likely, her team will consist of the following:

   a. Two RNs, an LPN, and unlicensed assistive personnel
   b. A licensed practical nurse and unlicensed assistive personnel
   c. A physician and unlicensed assistive personnel
   d. A dietary assistant and one unlicensed assistive personnel

500. A 72-year-old patient is recovering from abdominal surgery and asks the gerontological nurse about a new pink papular growth on his left ear. He wants it removed while he is in the hospital. Most likely this is:

   a. Herpes simplex 1
   b. Basal cell carcinoma
   c. Squamous cell carcinoma
   d. Malignant melanoma

501. Which of the following is a normal, age-related change related to the nervous system?

   a. A decrease in the number of functional neurons
   b. A steady loss of intellectual functioning
   c. Some loss of sensory perception
   d. An increase in nerve conduction fibers, causing greater sensitivity to pain

502. A 66-year-old man complains of fatigue, malaise, headaches, and an anterior neck mass. He is diagnosed with Hodgkin's lymphoma after many tests. One diagnostic finding in the cells of Hodgkin's lymphoma is:

   a. Philadelphia factor
   b. Cytokine-A
   c. Interferon B
   d. Reed-Sternberg cells

503. Older adults experiencing abdominal discomfort and altered bowel habits are generally diagnosed with which of the following conditions after normal gastrointestinal diagnostic testing?

   a. Crohn's disease
   b. Ulcerative colitis

    c. Spastic colon

    d. Irritable bowel disease

504. The most common outcome of poor compliance among older adults not following their medication regimen is:

    a. Overdosing

    b. Underdosing

    c. Family members using older adult's prescriptions

    d. Toxicity

505. You are bathing an 80-year-old man and you notice that his skin is wrinkled, thin, lax, and dry. This finding is related to which normal change of aging?

    a. Integumentary system changes

    b. Increases in elastin and subcutaneous fat

    c. An increase in the number of sweat and sebaceous glands

    d. Increased vascular flow to the skin

506. Older adults in respiratory failure often have a shallow and rapid breathing pattern or a slower respiratory rate. This further increases potential complications due to:

    a. Insufficient CO_2 removal

    b. Compensatory respiratory alkalosis

    c. Decreased lung recoil

    d. Increased vital capacity

507. Older patients on digoxin are most likely to experience the following side effect:

    a. Seeing halos around lights

    b. Tinnitus

    c. Confusion

    d. Anxiety

508. Loss of central vision due to macular degeneration is thought to be caused by trauma, aging, and infection. Symptoms of this eye problem include:

    a. Decreased color vision, distorted images, scotoma

    b. Decreased peripheral vision, diplopia, floaters

    c. Poor night vision, distorted images, loss of peripheral vision

    d. Astigmatism, myopia, distorted images

509. Older adults need to be questioned in depth regarding the following topic in the review of gastrointestinal systems:

    a. Abdominal bloating

    b. Bowel movement patterns

    c. Abdominal cramping

    d. Flatus

510. With the elderly, the appropriate index of measuring renal function is:

    a. BUN and creatinine
    b. Serum creatinine
    c. Creatinine clearance
    d. Tubular filtration rate

511. Many older adults in long-term care facilities experience urinary tract infections. Which organism is most often the pathology?

    a. Staphylococcus saprophyticus
    b. Streptococcus pneumoniae
    c. Escherichia coli
    d. Enterobacter

512. Eye examination for older adults should be referred to ophthalmologists and optometrists if the following are suspected:

    a. Cataracts and macular degeneration
    b. Glaucoma and risk of falling
    c. Glaucoma and vertigo
    d. Cerumen impaction and cataracts

513. All nurses have the potential to develop leadership skills. Some examples of leadership skills include:

    a. Managing the budget, orientation of new staff, and establishing safety policies
    b. Motivating staff, empowering others to lead, and creating a vision
    c. Motivating others, assisting all staff to be educated, and managing the schedule
    d. Registering all staff for educational programs, recommending staff become certified, and creating a strategic plan for the organization

514. Medicare and Medicaid legislation is an example of which of the following periods in U.S. health care history?

    a. 1940–1950
    b. 1960–1970
    c. 1980–1990
    d. 1990–2000

Answers

1. b. The presence of arcus senilus seen around the cornea
2. a. Graying of America
3. c. Manage disease, so it does not get worse.
4. b. Perform an electrocardiogram.
5. b. Increases contractility and decreases heart rate
6. b. Decreased cognitive status
7. c. Motivational theory
8. a. Decreased hydrogen/oxygen breakdown
9. c. Anorexia, nausea, and epigastric discomfort

10. c. Gout
11. c. Mission, philosophy, and goals of the organization
12. b. Septic arthritis secondary to gonorrhea and chlamydia
13. c. Cough
14. c. Transactional
15. d. Capsaicin cream
16. c. Cellulitis
17. d. Selected so that each member of a population has an equal probability of being included
18. a. Influenza vaccine
19. a. Compliance
20. a. B_{12} level
21. c. The older adult
22. d. To ensure the physical safety of the patient or other patients
23. c. Between 30 and 50 days posttransplant
24. c. Keep a daily written log of exercise and include type of exercise, time of exercise, and the intensity of exercise.
25. d. Institutional Review Board
26. b. Vitamin B_{12}
27. b. Medicare
28. d. Basal and bolus insulin
29. a. Anxiety
30. a. Protection from injury
31. d. Guarantee patient privacy.
32. a. Successful aging is dependent on the individual's developmental patterns throughout life.
33. a. Application of heat and/or cold—whichever is effective
34. b. Complications leading to death
35. c. Disorientation
36. d. Kaposi's sarcoma
37. b. ACE inhibitor
38. c. Decreased glomerular filtration rate
39. a. Prevent disease before it occurs
40. c. Osteoarthritis and osteoporosis
41. d. All of the above.
42. a. Periodontal disease
43. d. Encourage religious and spiritual practices at the end of life.
44. c. Evidence-based practice
45. d. Dizziness and tinnitus
46. b. Increase the brain's level of acetylcholine
47. a. Line of authority from the administrator to the unlicensed assistive personnel
48. c. Area Agencies on Aging
49. c. NSAIDs
50. b. Varies widely because of the loss of subcutaneous fat and muscle tissue
51. c. Heberden's nodes
52. b. AARP
53. a. Are nursing actions that will assist the patient to meet the identified goals

54. c. Beers Criteria
55. c. Decreased bladder capacity
56. b. "I am just too tired to do anything."
57. b. LDL should be less than 100.
58. c. Bathing
59. b. Detect disease at an earlier, more treatable stage.
60. b. Healthy People 2010
61. c. Kegel exercises
62. a. Excessive caffeine intake
63. b. Names a person for making health care decisions on behalf of the patient
64. a. Decreased diastolic blood pressure
65. c. Prednisone
66. d. Rosacea
67. a. Fewer killer T cells in the immunologic system
68. a. Increased technology
69. a. Carbohydrates
70. a. The "wear and tear" theory
71. b. Outcome, process, and structure
72. b. Lack of energy, fatigue, and malaise
73. d. Iron
74. b. Sign up for exercise class, get some sun, and do yoga.
75. b. "If there is no vitamin K in it, you can take it."
76. c. An elderly person may not exhibit outward signs of pain even when he or she is actually experiencing pain.
77. c. Malignancies and tuberculosis
78. b. OASIS Assessment
79. d. All of the above
80. a. Actinic keratosis
81. d. Keep up the good work!
82. b. Adverse effects of polypharmacy
83. d. Loss of elasticity of the lens
84. d. Gastrointestinal
85. c. Incompetent lower esophageal sphincter
86. c. Document them.
87. d. They cannot afford it.
88. c. Third-degree ankle sprain
89. a. Infection
90. c. 2.56–3.90 ng/mL
91. d. 85%
92. b. Recognize excellence in practice.
93. b. Delirium
94. a. Cherry angiomas, senile lentigines (liver spots), and skin tags
95. a. Written information describing the patient's desires for life-sustaining treatment
96. a. Vaginal atrophy and dryness
97. d. Smoking cessation
98. a. Active lifestyle
99. c. Renal dysfunction, neuropathy, and retinopathy

100. b. Optic neuritis
101. b. Developing cultural competence in the care of older adults
102. a. Cerebrovascular disease
103. a. Minimum Data Set
104. c. Holistic and caring
105. a. Medication errors, falls, skin breakdown, and infection rates
106. d. Hyperresonance
107. a. 24-hour ambulatory blood pressure monitoring
108. c. Methotrexate, hydroxychloroquine (Plaquenil)
109. c. Glaucoma
110. a. Orthopnea
111. d. Are you able to dress yourself?
112. b. Chronic lymphocytic leukemia
113. a. Measure an attribute consistently.
114. c. Cockcroft-Gault equation
115. b. Faces Scale
116. d. Constipation
117. d. Decreased muscle mass
118. b. Measuring the number of patients who had falls in their bedrooms
119. c. 1960s
120. c. 18.5 to 24.9
121. a. Fever and increased white blood cell count
122. a. Take extra time to adapt to the dim light before trying to find a seat
123. b. Assessment
124. a. Medicare
125. b. Pneumonia and atelectasis
126. b. A decrease in bladder muscle tone, which results in a lessened ability to postpone voiding.
127. b. Perform orthostatic blood pressure and pulse assessment.
128. c. 75%
129. c. Older American Resources and Services Assessment
130. d. Erythema, edema, blistering, ulceration
131. c. Rotator cuff tendonitis
132. c. Beneficence
133. b. Iron deficiency anemia
134. a. Presbycusis
135. b. Loss of sphincter control
136. b. To stabilize his vital signs and give fluid resuscitation
137. b. Airway protection
138. b. Nurses and health care professionals fail to detect problem alcohol use.
139. a. Cimetadine (Tagamet)
140. d. It was the first federal health care legislation to be broadly supported by the American Medical Association.
141. b. Continue for some years to come
142. b. Brain natriuretic peptide and complete chemistry profile
143. b. Once a day
144. b. Cardiovascular dysfunction
145. b. Genetic makeup, health behaviors, and availability of resources

146. a. Poor nutrition
147. d. Respite care
148. c. A number of chronic illnesses affect the sexual function of the elderly.
149. b. The patients can declare their desires regarding end-of-life care.
150. c. Acute exacerbations of their asthma
151. c. Hypothyroidism
152. c. She is of Asian ethnicity.
153. c. Inhibits the conversion of angiotensin I to angiotensin II
154. b. Depression, dementia, urinary function, and health literacy
155. d. All of the above
156. b. Paranoia
157. b. Noncompliant
158. b. An organized system of beliefs, practices, and rituals designed to foster closeness to a sacred reality
159. c. Have one nurse volunteer to develop and teach the wound care after learning it from a wound care consultant who is familiar with the procedure.
160. c. Failure to thrive
161. a. Aortic stenosis
162. b. Seborrheic keratosis
163. a. Measure an attribute consistently.
164. a. Increased levels of collagen
165. b. Polymyalgia rheumatica
166. a. Insulin will provide the quickest way to reach the optimum glycemic target for you.
167. d. Onset of delirium
168. c. Pharmacodynamics
169. b. Detached retina
170. d. Urge and stress
171. c. Good communication between the interdisciplinary team, patient, and family
172. d. Klebsiella pneumoniae
173. c. Condoms must be used to protect older adults against STDs.
174. b. Blurred vision and difficulty reading
175. b. Borderline blood cholesterol level
176. c. Inspection, palpation, percussion, and auscultation
177. c. Shortness of breath, fatigue, or epigastric discomfort
178. d. Assess Mr. L's preferred method of communication.
179. b. Sociological
180. a. Dysphagia
181. d. National Council of State Boards of Nursing
182. c. Both a and b
183. a. Is reversible/medications
184. d. A low-level type of care in which the emphasis is on doing to the patient rather that working with the patient
185. b. Hypothermia
186. b. Nuts, liver, and green leafy vegetables
187. d. Percocet
188. b. Quality improvement

189. c. "You have excess uric acid, which creates deposits of urate crystals in the soft tissue surrounding your peripheral joints."
190. c. Delirium
191. a. Right-sided infiltrate after chest X-ray
192. b. Cardiac output
193. c. Document why restraints are ordered, how they will be evaluated, and when they should be discontinued.
194. b. Medicaid
195. c. Anaphylaxis
196. d. Turn and reposition the patient every 1 to 2 hours.
197. b. The tool measures what it is intended to measure
198. a. Can be caused by bladder muscle weakness
199. a. Rigidity, bradykinesia, and tremors
200. b. Angina
201. b. Omnibus Budget Reconciliation Act
202. c. Increase
203. c. Increase in the production of estrogen
204. a. Arrange an appointment for him to see the physician.
205. c. 21%
206. c. Confusion
207. b. Herpes zoster
208. a. Free radicals
209. a. Family history
210. c. Minimal elevation in their white blood cell count
211. a. Dizziness
212. b. Bloodshot eye, photophobia, and irritation of eye
    Rationale: A corneal ulcer is manifested by complaints of eye irritation and photophobia as well as a bloodshot eye.
213. a. Cost-benefit analysis
214. d. Restorative
215. d. Seasonal allergies
216. d. Bronchoscopy
217. b. Nursing home or long-term care facility
218. b. Altered cognitive status
219. c. Pain and discomfort when urinating
220. b. Drug allergies
221. a. History of seizures
222. b. Pain
223. b. Peptic ulcer
224. b. Disorder of the basal ganglia that decreases ability to initiate movement
225. d. 75
226. a. Anticonvulsants
227. c. Decreased passage of oxygen from the alveoli to the blood
228. a. Assist with career goal accomplishment.
229. a. Bowing of limbs, hearing loss, and arthritis
230. b. Application of Anusol cream to the rectal area three times a day and after each bowel movement
231. a. State's Nurse Practice Act

232. b. Hyperthyroidism
233. b. A large secretory reserve in the main salivary glands
234. a. A continuing human need among older adults
235. d. Cognitive status assessment
236. a. Use less soap since it is drying, keep well hydrated, apply emollient cream
237. b. 50%
238. b. Urinary retention
239. b. Heart failure
240. a. Increased income
241. a. Delirium, urinary incontinence, falls, injuries, aspiration, emboli, and risk of restraint use
242. d. Moral/spiritual
243. d. 5 and 15 ug/ml
244. a. Urinary tract infection
245. c. Bony prominences
246. a. Widened bile duct
247. c. Focused history and physical exam and review of functional ability and medications
248. b. T cell deficiencies
     Rationale: With aging, changes in helper T cells' ability to function cause a decreased cellular immune response in older adults, which makes them more susceptible to infections.
249. c. Onychomycosis
250. b. Daytime napping of many older adults seems to compensate for night-time sleep disturbances.
251. b. Control group
252. a. Expectation that the problem is normal with aging, not wanting to bother anyone, high cost of drugs
253. b. A grayish arc surrounding the cornea
254. a. Infections and malignancies
255. a. Medicare
256. b. Some medications
257. c. Infections, smoking, medications
258. a. Have a high rate of exposure to latex such as with frequent dental procedures or surgeries
259. d. Previous history of a fall
260. d. Exercise the involved joints regularly.
261. a. Information disclosure, access to emergency services, and participation in treatment decisions
262. c. Helicobacter pylori
263. a. Regular exercise every day, losing weight, stopping smoking
264. d. 10 seconds
265. c. Diminished desires that occur as part of the aging process
266. b. Oxybutynin (Ditropan)
267. d. "There are medications that would dilate the small vessels in your hands and fingers, but these drugs would dilate other vessels, too, which could cause harm."
268. b. The safety culture of the institution

269. a. Cognitive status
270. a. Weakened vertebrae causing disk compression
271. d. Lupus erythematosus
272. c. Palliative
273. a. A redistribution of adipose tissue to the intra-abdominal region
274. d. "I have an order for a stool softener to put in my ostomy bag."
275. c. Decreased elasticity of vaginal epithelium
276. d. Provide information on patient's wishes at the end of life.
277. c. The Joint Commission
278. a. The patient develops confusion or exhibits a change in mental status.
279. a. Primary
280. a. 3 months ago
281. a. Biological
282. d. Collaboration
283. a. Renal dialysis every other day
284. d. Catecholamine surges impacting circadian rhythm
285. c. Beta blockers
286. c. Rheumatoid arthritis
287. b. 20%
288. c. Katz Index
289. c. Dizziness and lightheadedness
290. b. Medicaid
291. d. Cerumen impaction
292. d. Hips and knees
293. b. Corn
294. c. Quantitative research
295. a. Fine needle biopsy
296. c. Provide patients the opportunity to develop advanced directives.
297. c. Medications
298. b. Discomfort, hurting, aching
299. c. Complete blood count
300. a. Primary
301. a. Intake and output, mucous membrane moisture, and urine specific gravity
302. c. Taking it no more than once every 24 hours
303. c. Provides information for the distribution of financial assets
304. c. An aged person has a longer story to tell.
305. a. NSAIDs
306. c. Psychological
307. b. Decreasing osteoblast function
308. c. T cells
    Rationale: Older adults experience an overall decline in immunological capabilities.
309. c. Polypharmacy
310. b. Excessive urination, high blood glucose levels, increased thirst
311. c. Pneumonia
312. b. A duodenal ulcer
313. a. Orthopnea
314. b. Qualitative research

315. d. Rising Medicare costs
316. b. Autoimmune disorders
317. b. Acetaminophen (Tylenol)
318. b. Iron deficiency anemia
319. c. Modification of hypothalamic function
320. b. Zoloft
321. c. Fewer areoli
322. c. Metabolic syndrome
323. b. Secondary
324. a. Urinary tract infection
325. d. Helper T cells
326. b. Sociological
327. b. Gait disturbance, dizziness, impaired concentration
328. d. Sensorineural and conductive hearing loss
329. a. Live and die with dignity
330. b. Polyuria, erectile dysfunction, increased frequency
331. b. Lack of standards
332. a. The entire staff is involved in any decision making regarding the change.
333. c. Businesses
334. a. High-fiber diet and prevention of constipation
335. d. Depression, anxiety, sleep disturbance
336. d. Unequal pupillary constriction in response to light
337. d. Nursing process
338. a. Pregnant women, infants, people who are immunocompromised
339. a. Headache, seizures, vomiting
340. b. Benadryl
341. d. Arrange a psychiatric consult for evaluation of her depression and treatment.
342. b. A natural extension of life
343. a. Appointment of Social Security beneficiaries
344. a. Sister Callista Roy
345. c. Hodgkin's disease
346. b. Secondary
347. d. 100%
348. c. Hashimoto's disease
349. a. Fatigue
350. d. Passive neglect
351. a. Organ system degeneration
352. a. Salt and sugar
353. a. Blood pressure and pulse while lying, sitting, and standing
354. a. Dislocation of the prosthesis
355. a. Integumentary system changes
356. c. Shortness of breath, a change in her cough pattern, and fatigue
357. d. The family's grieving process is complete.
358. b. Delirium
359. b. Risedronate (Actonel)
360. b. Mental status for confusion or disorientation
361. b. Systolic blood pressure decrease of 20 mmHg and a diastolic blood pressure decrease of 10 mmHg after a position change

362. c. American Nurses Association
363. c. A decline
364. c. NSAIDs, steroids, diuretics
365. d. Balding in patches
366. b. Is a progressive conductive hearing loss that commonly occurs with age
367. a. Heartburn after a big meal or when lying supine
368. c. Explain to Mr. Carter that this is a normal age-related change that occurs in the eye.
369. b. Stress/Kegel exercises
370. a. Using an active listening approach to communication
371. c. Open questioning, acknowledging, and summarizing
372. a. Increased body fat
373. d. Dame Cicely Saunders
374. d. Dorothy Orem
375. c. Decreased respiratory muscle strength, decreased airway and lung compliance
376. c. Dementia
377. c. Tertiary
378. c. 300–400 ng/dL
379. d. Motivation, identification of staff feelings, and emotional self-management
380. a. Medicare Part A
381. d. Bone reabsorption causes the bone to lose calcium and decreases the ability to produce material for the bone matrix.
382. a. Interleukin 6 and tumor necrosis factor alpha
383. a. Posttraumatic stress disorder
384. a. Muscular pain from overuse
385. a. Polypharmacy
386. d. Transactional leadership
387. d. The glomerular filtration rate in the kidneys increases with age, resulting in an increase in the excretion of drugs.
388. b. Temporal arteritis
389. b. Optimal patient outcomes, access to services, and cost-effectiveness
390. d. All of the above
391. b. Onychomycosis
392. a. Most people become edentulous (lose their teeth).
393. a. Absorption
394. c. Central vision loss
395. c. Neutropenia, anemia, and thrombocytopenia
396. a. There is a very small amount of radioactivity emitted after treatment.
397. b. The movement of drugs within the body
398. c. Improved development and access to diagnostic tests and technology
399. c. Erythropoietin (Epogen)
400. c. Spiritual assessment
401. a. Smoking since the age of 18
402. b. Hildegarde Peplau
403. c. A "good death"
404. b. Essential tremor
405. c. Gout

406. d. Memantine (Namenda)
407. c. Hypermagnesemia
408. b. Hypothyroidism
409. a. The Geriatric Depression Scale
410. a. Six Sigma
411. d. The patient becomes short of breath when ambulating to the bathroom.
412. b. Decreased sensitivity to insulin
413. b. Alcohol use
414. b. Evidence-based research
415. b. Electrolyte imbalance
416. a. Stop eating grapefruit or grapefruit juice.
417. b. Drug sensitivity
418. c. Residual volume decreases with age.
419. c. Performance and continued improvement in care
420. a. Presbycusis
421. c. S_4
422. c. Changes in behavior, fatigue, and loss of appetite
423. a. Tremor, palpitations, and proximal weakness
424. c. The heart valves stiffen and become thicker.
425. a. Keep the wound open to air during the day and covered with wet to dry dressing at night, make sure her position and adult brief are changed frequently, discuss plans for nursing home placement.
426. a. Nursing grand theory
427. a. Physical
428. b. Non-Hodgkin's disease
429. c. Yes, there is a relationship between family history and dementia.
430. d. Medigap
431. b. Hypothermia
432. c. Delayed gastric emptying
433. b. Increased receptor affinity
434. b. Encouraging a good relationship between the patient and the health care provider
435. d. 50 and 100 ml
436. c. Benign paroxysmal positional vertigo
437. c. Alendronate (Fosomax)
438. b. Following the organization's policies and procedures to generate high-quality care
439. b. Shared knowledge with patient, anticipated patient needs, and customized care
440. c. Metabolic syndrome
441. a. Physical
442. a. Can be caused by bladder muscle weakness
443. c. Brain tumor
444. c. End-of-life care often provides an opportunity to help patients complete important psychological and developmental tasks of aging.
445. b. Male gender, obesity, older than 65 yrs
446. d. HMOs
447. c. High bulk in diet, exercise routines

448. b. Rule out delirium and depression as contributors to altered cognitive function.
449. a. Communicator, visionary role model, and change maker
450. c. 1,000,000
451. b. Deep vein thrombosis
452. d. Cataract
453. a. Polypharmacy
454. b. A decrease in bladder muscle tone results in a lessened ability to postpone voiding.
455. d. Respiratory
456. d. Osteoporosis
457. c. Chronic myelogenous leukemia
458. d. Folstein Mini-Mental State Examination
459. a. Ombudsman
460. d. All of the above
461. c. Decreased metabolic clearance of cortisol
462. c. Active neglect
463. d. Pain
464. b. Egg albumin
465. c. Actinic keratosis
466. c. Perform a needs survey of the staff to determine what they want to gain regarding leadership skills.
467. b. Identifying specific self-care deficits
468. c. Metformin (Glucophage)
469. b. Decreased liver function
470. c. Increased pH
471. b. Medicaid
472. c. Urinary frequency, urgency, and nocturia
473. b. 70 to 75 mmHg
474. a. 24-hour recall
475. a. Is reversible
476. a. Bell's Palsy
477. a. Power
478. b. Blurred vision and night vision loss
479. b. Periodontitis
480. a. Metformin (Glucophage)
481. b. Fluoxetine (Prozac)
482. c. Intermittent claudication
483. b. Psychological
484. b. Memory loss, mood changes, changes in personality
485. b. Spiritual
486. a. Confusion, tremors, weakness, diaphoresis
487. a. Changed Medicare from being a private insurer to managed care
488. a. Either performance or capacity
489. a. A functional assessment is used to evaluate the overall ability of older adults to independently complete their activities of daily living.
490. a. Registered nurse, licensed practical nurses, and unlicensed assistive personnel
491. d. Hip

492. a. Brenner and Wrubel
493. b. Amitriptyline (Elavil)
494. a. Prostate gland hypertrophy
495. d. Both b and c.
496. d. Roast beef, peanut butter sandwiches, and spinach salad
497. a. Spirituality may provide a framework within which older adults search for meaning and purpose in life.
498. b. Thrombotic cerebrovascular accident
499. b. A licensed practical nurse and unlicensed assistive personnel
500. b. Basal cell carcinoma
501. a. A decrease in the number of functional neurons
502. d. Reed-Sternberg cells
503. d. Irritable bowel disease
504. b. Underdosing
505. a. Integumentary system changes
506. a. Insufficient CO_2 removal
507. c. Confusion
508. a. Decreased color vision, distorted images, scotoma
509. b. Bowel movement patterns
510. c. Creatinine clearance
511. c. Escherichia coli
512. a. Cataracts and macular degeneration
513. b. Motivating staff, empowering others to lead, and creating a vision
514. b. 1960–1970

Index

AAA. *See* Area agencies on aging
AARP. *See* American Association of
    Retired Persons
Abdellah and colleagues nursing theory, 21
Abdomen assessment, 34
Absorption, drug, 127
Abuse, 136–138
Accreditation, 171
Acculturation, 18
Activity theory, 22
Acute and chronic physical illnesses,
    83–110
  anemia, 93–94
  angina and myocardial infarction (MI),
    86–88
  cancer, 96–98
  cerebral vascular accidents (CVAs),
    104–105
  congestive heart failure (CHF), 84–86
  diabetes mellitus (DM), 100–101
  ear diseases, 110
  eye diseases, 108–109
  gastroesophageal reflux disease, 92–93
  HIV/AIDS, 101–102
  hypertension, 83–84
  influenza, 90–91
  obstructive airway disease, 92
  osteoarthritis and degenerative joint
    disease, 98–99
  osteoporosis, 99–100
  Parkinson's disease (PD), 102–104
  peripheral vascular disease (PVD),
    88–89
  pneumonia, 89–90
  sexually transmitted diseases (STDs),
    94–96
  transient ischemic attacks (TIAs),
    104–105
  tuberculosis, 91–92
  urinary tract infections, 94

AD. *See* Alzheimer's disease
Adam's equity theory, 23
Advanced directives, 78–80, 173
Adverse reactions, 128–129
Advocacy, 139–140
Ageism and myths of aging, 14–17
Aging changes, normal, 37–41
  cardiovascular system, 37
  gastrointestinal system, 38–39
  integumentary system, 38
  neurological system, 41
  peripheral vascular system, 37
  respiratory system, 38
  sensory system, 40–41
  sexual/reproductive system, 40
  urinary system, 39
Aging in place, 62, 68
Aging population, 13–28
  ageism and myths of aging, 15–17
  aging theories, 21–22
  categories, 14
  communication with, 23–26
  cultural sensitivity to, 18–19
  demographics of, 13–14
  family theory, 22–23
  gerontological nursing, 27–28
  motivational theory, 23
  nursing theories, 19–21
  teaching-learning theories and
    principles, 26–27
Aging theories, 21–22
AIDS (Acquired Immune Deficiency
    Syndrome), 101–102
Alcohol use, 44–47
ALFs. *See* Assisted living facilities
Alternative care, 55–57
Alzheimer's disease (AD), 119–121
American Association of Retired Persons
    (AARP), 139–140
American Geriatrics Society, 28

American Nurses Association, 27, 174
American Nurses Credentialing Center
  (ANCC), 5
American Society of Aging, 28
ANCC. *See* American Nurses
  Credentialing Center
Anemia, 93–94
Angina and myocardial infarction (MI),
  86–88
ANNC certification, 5
Area agencies on aging (AAA), 141
Assessment, 29–41
  health history, 29–32
  normal aging changes, 37–41
  physical, 32–36
Assisted living facilities (ALFs), 67

Barriers to health promotion, 44
Beneficence, 173
Benefit to society of older adults, 15
Benner and Wrubel nursing theory, 21
Biological theories of aging, 21
Black licorice, 55
Blood pressure, 32–33
Body mass index (BMI), 32
Breast cancer, 98

Cancer, 96–97
Cardiac illnesses, 83–89
Cardiovascular system, 37
Care, environments of. *See* Environments
  of care
Caregivers, 66
Carotid endarterectomy procedures, 105
Cascara sagrada, 55
Cataracts, 108
CCRCs. *See* Continuing care retirement
  communities
Centenarians, 17
Centers for Medicare and Medicaid
  Services, 171
Cerebral vascular accidents (CVAs),
  104–105
Certification exam, 1–5
  content outline, 2–3
  format, 2
  hints for test takers, 5
  number of questions, 3
  overview, 1
  results, 4
  scheduling, 3–4
  time allowed, 3
  See also Question dissection and analysis
Certification validity period, 5

Chemical restraints, 60
CHF. *See* Congestive heart failure
Chlamydia trachomates, 95–96
Chronic illnesses. *See* Acute and chronic
  physical illnesses
Claudication, intermittent, 88
Code of Ethics for Nurses, 174
Cognitive and psychological disorders,
  111–124
  delirium, 112–113, 122–123
  dementia, 112–113, 119–122
  depression, 112–118
  suicide, 118–119
Cognitive status, 31
Cognitive teaching-learning theories, 26
Communication with older adults, 23–25,
  78
Community-based services and resources,
  65–66
Compliance issues, medication, 129
Complimentary care, 55–57
Conditions experienced by older adults, 9
Confusion, acute, 122
Congestive heart failure (CHF), 84–86
Conscience incompetence, 19
Conscious competence, 19
Constipation, 39
Constructivist theories, 26
Continuing care retirement communities
  (CCRCs), 67–68
Continuity theory, 22
Cost-benefit analysis, 170
*Crossing the Quality Chasm: A New Health
  System for the 21st Century*, 171
Cultural competence, 18–19
Cultural shifts in health care, 18
CVAs. *See* Cerebral vascular accidents

Death, readiness for, 17
Death and dying, 71–82
  advanced directives, 78–80
  end-of-life care, 71–78
  grieving, 81–82
  hospice and palliative care, 80
  widowhood, 81–82
Decubitis ulcers, 105–108, 109
Deep vein thrombosis, 89
Degenerative joint disease, 98–99
Delirium, 31, 112–113, 122–123
Dementia, 112–113, 119–122
Department of Veterans Affairs (VA), 166
Depression, 16, 112–118, 134
Diabetes mellitus (DM), 100–101, 135
Disease management, 44

Diseases. *See* Acute and chronic physical illnesses; *specific diseases*
Disengagement theory, 22
DM. *See* Diabetes mellitus
Driving, 63–64
Drug absorption, 127
Drug interactions, 128–129
Drugs. *See* Medication
Drugs, elimination of, 128
Durable power of attorney for health care, 79–80
Dying. *See* Death and dying

Ear diseases, 110
Eldercare Locator, 141
Elder neglect and abuse, 136–138
Elimination of drugs, 128
Endocrine problems, 100–101
End-of-life care, 17, 71–78, 173
    physical, 72–74
    psychological, 72–75, 76
    social, 75
    spiritual, 75–78
Environments of care, 59–69
    community-based services and resources, 65–66
    homeless elders, 68–69
    hypo- and hyperthermia, 62
    relocation, 62–63
    residential facilities, 66–68
    safety and security issues, 59–60
    territoriality and personal space, 64–65
    transportation, 63–64
    use of restraints, 60–61
Equity theory, Adam's, 23
Erickson's theory of integrity vs. despair, 22
Ethical principles of geriatric nursing, 173–174
Ethnogerontology, 18
Exam, certification. *See* Certification exam
Exam, practice, 3
Exam preparation strategies. *See* Certification exam; Question dissection and analysis
Exercise, 48
Eye diseases, 108–109

Faces Pain Scale, 132
Failure to thrive (FTT), 47–48
Falls, 59–61
Family theory of aging, 22–23
Fecal impaction, 39
Fecal incontinence, 39

Fingernail growth assessment, 33
Five Rights of Delegation, 173
FTT. *See* Failure to thrive
Functional Status Assessment, 171

Gastroesophageal reflux disease, 92–93
Gastrointestinal problems, 92–93
Gastrointestinal system, 38–39
Genetics, 17
Genital herpes, 95–96
Genitourinary assessment, 34
Genitourinary problems, 94–96
Geriatric nursing, defined, 27
Geriatric nursing, scope and standards of, 169–176
    evidence-based practice, 175
    leadership, 169–170
    legal and ethical issues, 173–174
    management, 170
    organizational concepts, 172
    professional development, 172–173
    quality improvement, 171–172
    research, 174–175
Gerontic nursing, defined, 27
Gerontological certification exam. *See* Certification exam
Gerontological nursing, defined, 27–28
Gerontological Society of America, 28
Gerotranscendance, Thorstam's theory of, 22
Ginger, 55
Ginko bilboa, 55
Ginseng, 55
Glaucoma, 109
Glucosamine, 55
Gonorrhea, 95–96
Good death, 71
Graying of America. *See* Aging population
Grieving, 81–82

Hair growth and nails assessment, 33
Head and neck assessment, 33–34
Health care delivery systems, 140
Health history, 29–32
Health Insurance and Portability Act, 173
Health literacy, 27
Health policy issues. *See* Organizational and health policy issues
Health promotion, 43–58
    alcohol use, 44–47
    alternative and complimentary care, 55–57
    barriers to, 44
    exercise, 48

Health promotion (*continued*)
immunization, 51–53
levels of prevention, 43–44
nutrition and hydration, 47–50
sleep, 48–51, 54
smoking, 47
Health promotion activities, 23
Hearing, 41
Hearing aids, 110
Heart assessment, 34
Heat stroke, 62
Height measurement, 32
Hematological problems, 93–94
Henderson nursing theory, 21
Herbal medications/supplements,
55–57, 125
Herpes, 95–96
Herzberg's hygienic needs theory, 23
HIV (Human Immunodeficiency Virus),
101–102
Home, living at, 64–65
Homeless elders, 68–69
Hospice, 80
Human papilloma virus, 95–96
Hydration, 47–48
Hygiene, personal, 17
Hygienic needs theory, Hertzberg's, 23
Hypertension, 32–33, 83–84
Hyperthermia, 62
Hypothermia, 62

Illnesses, acute and chronic. *See* Acute
and chronic physical illnesses
Immunization, 51–55
Immunologic problems, 101–102
Impaction, fecal, 39
Incontinence, 17, 39–40
Influenza, 90–91
Informed consent, 174
Insurance, long-term care, 165–166
Integrity versus despair, theory of, 22
Integumentary system, 38
Intellectual activity, 16
Intermittent claudication, 88

Joint Commission, 171–172
Jung's theory of self-realization, 22

Katz Index, 31
Kegel exercises, 40
King nursing theory, 21
Kolberg's theory of self-transcendence, 22
Kubler-Ross, stages of grieving, 81
Kyphosis, 100

Laboratory tests, 34–36
Leadership, 169–170
Legal issues in geriatric nursing,
173–175
Leininger nursing theory, 21
Levels of prevention, 43–46
Licorice, black, 55
Living wills, 79
Longevity, 14
Long-term care insurance, 165–166
Lungs assessment, 34

Management, nursing, 170
Maslow's theory of self-actualization, 22
McClelland's motivational theory, 23
McGregor's X-Y theory, 23
MDS. *See* Minimum Data Set
Medicaid, 79, 163–165
Medical power of attorney, 79–80
Medicare, 68, 79, 141–162
fee-for-service plans, 163
Managed Care, 162–163
Medication, 125–129
adverse reactions and side effects,
128–129
compliance issues, 129
pharmacokenetics and
pharmacodynamics, 126–128
Medications, herbal, 55–57, 125
Medigap, 162
Memory loss. *See* dementia
Memory loss, normal, 120
Metabolic problems, 100–101
MI. *See* Myocardial infarction
Mini-Cog, 31–32, 121
Minimum Data Set (MDS), 67
Mistreatment, 136–138
Mnemonics, 10
Moral/spiritual theory of aging, 22
Motivational theory, 23
Musculoskeletal problems, 98–100
Musculoskeletal system assessment, 34
Myocardial infarction (MI), 86–88
Myths of aging, 15–17, 26

National Center for Cultural Competence,
19
National Council of State Boards of
Nursing (NCSBN), 173
National Council on Aging (NCOA), 140
National Gerontological Nursing
Organization, 28
National Patient Safety Goals, 172
NCOA. *See* National Council on Aging

NCSBN. *See* National Council of State Boards of Nursing

Neglect, 136–138

Neisseria gonorrhorae (gonorrhea), 95–96

Neuman nursing theory, 21

Neurological problems, 102–105

Neurological system, 41

Neutraseuticals, 55–57

Nightingale nursing theory, 19

Nonmalfeasance, 174

Nonprescriptions, 125

Normal aging changes. *See* Aging changes, normal

Nurse Practice Act, 173

Nursing theories, 19–21

Nutrition, 47–50

OASIS. *See* Outcome and assessment information set

O'Brien's Spiritual Assessment Scale, 77

Obstructive airway disease, 92

Older adults. *See* Aging population

Older American Resources and Services Assessment, 171

Older Americans Act of 1965, 141

Ombudsman, 173

Omnibus Budget Reconciliation Act of 1987, 61

Orem nursing theory, 21

Organizational and health policy issues, 139–167
   advocacy, 139–140
   health care delivery systems, 140
   long-term care insurance, 165–166
   Medicaid, 163–165
   Medicare and Medigap, 141–163
   Older Americans Act of 1965, 141
   reimbursement, 140–141
   veteran's benefits, 166

Osteoarthritis, 98–99

Osteoporosis, 99–100

Outcome and assessment information set (OASIS), 65

Over-the-counter (OTC) medications, 125

Pain, 131–134

Palliative care, 71–72, 78, 80

Parkinson's disease (PD), 102–104, 119

Patient Self-Determination Act, 79

PD. *See* Parkinson's disease

Peplau nursing theory, 21

Peripheral vascular disease (PVD), 88–89

Peripheral vascular system, 37

Personal hygiene, 17

Personal issues, unresolved, 72, 75

Personality, alteration of, 15

Personal space, 64–65

Pharmacodynamics, 126–128

Pharmacokenetics, 126–128

Physical assessment, 32–36

Physical illnesses. *See* Acute and chronic physical illnesses

Physical restraints, 60

Pneumonia, 89–90

Polypharmacy, 125

Power of attorney, 79–80

PPOs. *See* Preferred provider organizations

PPS. *See* Prospective payment system

Practice exam, 3

Preferred provider organizations (PPOs), 163

Presbycusis, 110

Prescriptions, 125

Prevention, levels of, 43–46

Primary prevention, 43–44

Prospective payment system (PPS), 163

Prostate cancer, 97

Psychological disorders. *See* Cognitive and psychological disorders

Psychological theories of aging, 22

Pulse, 32

PVD. *See* Peripheral vascular disease

Question dissection and analysis, 7–12
   preparation strategies, 7–8
   question types, 9
   red flag problems, 9
   strategies for, 9–12

Reimbursement, 140–141

Religion. *See* Spirituality

Relocation, 62–63

Research, nursing, 174–175

Residential facilities, 66–68

Respiration, 32

Respiratory problems, 89–92

Respiratory system, 38

Respite care, 66

Restraints, 60–61

Right-to-die laws, 173

Rogers nursing theory, 21

Roy and Andrews nursing theory, 21

Safety and security issues, 59–60

Saw palmetto, 55

Scope and standards of geriatric nursing. *See* Geriatric nursing, scope and standards of

Screening, 44–46
Secondary prevention, 44–46
Security issues, 59–60
Self-actualization, Mazlow's theory of, 22
Self-realization, Jung's theory of, 22
Self-transcendence, Kolberg's theory of, 22
Sensory system, 40–41
Sexuality, 16, 133–136
Sexually transmitted diseases (STDs), 94–96
Sexual/reproductive system, 40
Side effects of drugs, 128–129
Six Sigma, 172
Skilled nursing facilities (SNFs), 66–67
Skin assessment, 33
Sleep, 48–51, 54
Smell, sense of, 41
Smoking, 38, 47
SNFs. *See* Skilled nursing facilities
Sociological theories of aging, 22
Spiritual assessment scales, 77
Spirituality, 75–78
Stages of grieving, 81
STDs. *See* Sexually transmitted diseases
St. John's wort, 55
Stoll's Spiritual Assessment Guide, 77
Strokes, 104–105
Suicide, 118–119
Supplements, herbal, 55–57, 125
Syphilis, 95–96

Tasks, unfinished, 72, 75
Taste, sense of, 41
Teaching-learning theories and principles, 26–27
Temperature, 32
Territoriality, 64–65
Tertiary prevention, 44
Test, certification. *See* Certification exam
Thrombosis, deep vein, 89

TIAs. *See* Transient ischemic attacks
Toenail growth assessment, 33
Tornstam's theory of gerotranscendence, 22
Transactional leadership, 169
Transformational leadership, 169–170
Transient ischemic attacks (TIAs), 104–105
Translocation syndrome, 62–63
Transportation, 63–64
Treponema palladium (syphilis), 95–96
Tuberculosis, 91–92

Ulcers, 109
Unconscious competence, 19
Unconscious incompetence, 18
Unfinished tasks, 72, 75
Uniform Benefits Package, veterans, 166
Unresolved personal issues, 72, 75
Urinary incontinence, 39–40
Urinary system, 39
Urinary tract infections, 94
Utilitarianism, 174

VA. *See* Department of Veterans Affairs
Veracity, 174
Veteran's benefits, 166
Veterans' Health Care Eligibility Reform Act of 1996, 166
Vision, 40–41
Visual Analogue Scale (VAS), 132
Vital signs, 32
Vitamins, 55

Watson nursing theory, 21
Weight measurement, 32
Western biomedical model of health care, 18
Widowhood, 81–82
Wills, 79–80

X-Y theory, McGregor's, 23

SPRINGER PUBLISHING COMPANY

Home Health Care Provider
A Guide to Essential Skills
Emily Prieto, MBA, LSW

This book is designed to foster quality care to home care recipients. It is written for companions, home health aides, and other caregivers who deliver nonmedical home care. Prieto provides information, tips, and techniques on personal care routines as well as additional responsibilities that are often necessary in this work, including home safety and maintenance, meal planning, errand running, caring for couples, and making use of recreational time. Going beyond standard nurses' aide training manuals, the book focuses on the psychosocial needs of home care recipients, stressing the need to maintain the house as a home and sustaining the recipient's way of life throughout caregiving situations. Prieto stresses interpersonal skills that benefit recipient and caregiver, creating a systematic, easy-to-follow plan for delivering quality service and maintaining, or improving, quality of life.

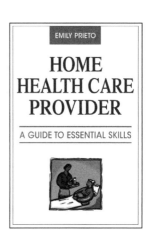

Contents:
- Attitudes of Aging
- Aging at Home
- The Companion Home Care Provider
- Interpersonal Skills and Communications
- Common Conditions & Diseases of the Aging Body
- The Terminally Ill Client
- Caring for Couples
- About Activities
- Planning and Preparing Meals
- Home Safety and Household Management
- Legal and Financial
- Planning for Placement

2008 · 248 pp · 978-0-8261-2852-2 · softcover

11 West 42nd Street, New York, NY 10036-8002 • Fax: 212-941-7842
Order Toll-Free: 877-687-7476 • Order Online: www.springerpub.com

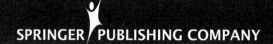
Geriatric Nursing

Growth of a Specialty

Priscilla Ebersole, PhD, RN, FAAN
Theris A. Touhy, ND, APRN, BC

Learn the history of the development of geriatric nursing as a specialty, as well as the current state of geriatric nursing, from the stories of pioneers in this field. Through the history of those who laid the foundations for the profession, to the geriatric nurse leaders who continue the specialty today, see first-hand how geriatric nursing began, evolved, and continues to flourish.

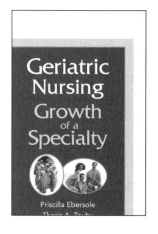

Covering the scope of the specialty:

- How to become a geriatric nurse
- Geriatric nursing organizations and publications
- Standards of practice
- Certification and licensure
- Future directions

This text provides both inspirational stories of nursing and practical information on how you can find resources, develop ideas, and access research in order to become a successful geriatric nurse.

Partial Contents

History and Development of Geriatric Nursing • Geriatric Nurse Pioneers and Their Contributions • Nurses in Action: The Second Generation • Geriatric Nurse Leaders Today • Recognition of Geriatric Care as a Specialty Practice • Geriatric Nursing Organizations and Affiliates • Educational Programs and Publications for Geriatric and Gerontological Nurses • Nursing Research and Geriatric Care • Elements of Attracting Nurses to the Field • Nursing and the Future Care of the Aged: Possibilities and Opportunities

2006 · 304pp · 978-0-8261-2649-8 · softcover

11 West 42nd Street, New York, NY 10036-8002 • Fax: 212-941-7842
Order Toll-Free: 877-687-7476 • Order Online: www.springerpub.com

The Encyclopedia of Elder Care

The Comprehensive Resource on Geriatric and Social Care
Second Edition

Elizabeth A. Capezuti, PhD, RN, FAAN
Eugenia L. Siegler, MD, FACP
Mathy D. Mezey, EdD, RN, FAAN, Editors

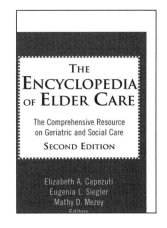

"This encyclopedia is a compendium that reflects on that new growth in leadership and knowledge in the field. Drs. Capezuti, Siegler, and Mezey are to be congratulated for their remarkable ability to assemble the most outstanding researchers, clinicians, and policymakers to author these informative and useful chapters. With the 'agewave' upon us, inconceivable numbers of older adults will be seeking appropriate, humane, quality care that is data-driven and responsive to the best information in hand. This encyclopedia provides that best information and creates a new baseline from which professions in aging will continue to thrive and grow."

—Terry Fulmer, Dean, College of Nursing, New York University

Features new to this second edition:
- More extensive use of online resources for further information on topics
- Thoroughly updated entries and references
- Inclusion of current research in geriatrics reflecting evidence-based practice
- New topics, including Assisted Living, Nursing Home Managed Care, Self-Neglect, Environmental Modifications (Home & Institution), Technology, Neuropsychological Assessment, Psychoactive Medications, Pain—Acute and Chronic

Still the only reference of its kind, the **Encyclopedia of Elder Care** will prove to be an indispensable tool for all professionals in the field of aging, such as nurses, physicians, social workers, counselors, health administrators, and more.

2007 · 950pp · 978-0-8261-0259-1 · hardcover

11 West 42nd Street, New York, NY 10036-8002 • Fax: 212-941-7842
Order Toll-Free: 877-687-7476 • Order Online: www.springerpub.com

SPRINGER PUBLISHING COMPANY

Evidence-Based Geriatric Nursing Protocols for Best Practice

Third Edition

Elizabeth Capezuti, PhD, RN, FAAN
DeAnne Zwicker, MS, APRN, BC
Mathy Mezey, EdD, RN, FAAN
Terry T. Fulmer, PhD, RN, FAAN, Editors
Deanna Gray-Miceli, DNSc, APRN,
Associate Editor
Malvina Kluger, Managing Editor

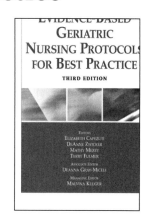

"This third edition holds the promise of bringing yet another level of depth and sophistication to understanding the best practices for assessment, interventions, and anticipated outcomes in our care of older adults. **Evidence-Based Geriatric Nursing Protocols for Best Practice** *is intended to bring the most current, evidence-based protocols known to experts in geriatric nursing to the audience of students, both graduate and undergraduate, practitioners at the staff level from novice to expert, clinicians in specialty roles (educators, care managers, and advanced practice nurses), and nursing leaders of all levels."*

—from the Preface by **Susan Bowar-Ferres,** PhD, RN, CNAA-BC
Senior Vice President & Chief Nursing Officer
New York University Hospitals Center

This is the third, thoroughly revised and updated edition of the book formerly entitled **Geriatric Nursing Protocols for Best Practice.** The protocols address key clinical conditions and circumstances likely to be encountered by a hospital nurse caring for older adults. They represent "best practices" for acute care of the elderly as developed by nursing experts around the country as part of the *Hartford Foundation's Nurses Improving Care to the Hospitalized Elderly project (NICHE).*

This third edition includes 17 revised and updated chapters and more than 15 new topics including critical care, diabetes, hydration, oral health care, palliative care, and substance abuse.

2007 · 736pp · 978-0-8261-1103-6 · hardcover

11 West 42nd Street, New York, NY 10036-8002 • Fax: 212-941-7842
Order Toll-Free: 877-687-7476 • Order Online: www.springerpub.com